MEDICAL TECHNOLOGY MANAGEMENT PRACTICE

ABOUT THE AUTHOR

Anthony Y. K. Chan graduated in Electrical Engineering (B.Sc. Hon.) from the University of Hong Kong in 1979, completed a M.Sc. degree in Engineering from the same university and worked as an electrical project engineer. He completed a Master of Engineering Degree (M.Eng.) in Clinical Engineering from the University of British Columbia in Canada in 1987. He also holds a Certificate in Hospital Services Management from the Canadian Hospital Association. Anthony was the manager and director of biomedical engineering in a number of Canadian acute care hospitals. He is currently the Program Head of the Biomedical Engineering Technology Program at the British Columbia Institute of Technology. He is a professional engineer and a certified clinical engineer.

MEDICAL TECHNOLOGY MANAGEMENT PRACTICE

By

ANTHONY Y. K. CHAN

Biomedical Engineering Technology
British Columbia Institute of Technology
Burnaby, British Columbia, Canada

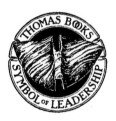

CHARLES C THOMAS • PUBLISHER, LTD.
Springfield • Illinois • U.S.A.

Published and Distributed Throughout the World by

CHARLES C THOMAS • PUBLISHER, LTD.
2600 South First Street
Springfield, Illinois 62704

© 2003 by CHARLES C THOMAS • PUBLISHER, LTD.

ISBN 0-398-07414-3 (hard)
ISBN 0-398-07415-1 (paper)

Library of Congress Catalog Card Number: 2003044044

With THOMAS BOOKS *careful attention is given to all details of manufacturing
and design. It is the Publisher's desire to present books that are satisfactory as to their
physical qualities and artistic possibilities and appropriate for their particular use.*
THOMAS BOOKS *will be true to those laws of quality that assure a good name
and good will.*

Printed in the United States of America
SM-R-3

Library of Congress Cataloging-in-Publication Data

Chan, Anthony Y. K.
    Medical technology management practice / by Anthony Y. K. Chan.
        p. cm.
    Includes index.
    ISBN 0-398-07414-3 (hbk.) -- ISBN 0-398-07415-1 (pbk.)
    1. Medical technology. 2. Medical innovations. I. Title.

R855.3.C477 2003
610'.28--dc21

2003044044

To my wife Elaine
and
my parents, Chung Ping Chan and How Fong Chan

PREFACE

With continuous rapid advancement, technology has infiltrated into all parts of everyday life. Modern health care delivery and medicine are increasingly dependent on technology in the diagnosis and mitigation of illnesses, in disease prevention, and in health promotion. Medical technology is one of the driving forces in shaping the direction of health care. However, it is also a primary factor for the escalating cost in the health care delivery system. For these reasons, it is important for managers to master the arts and methodologies in medical technology management so that technology can be used appropriately, effectively, and efficiently.

This book studies the medical technology life cycle from the user's perspective, starting from technology acquisition to disposal. It takes a practical approach to analyze medical technology management in clinical settings. General practices are described throughout the book, concepts are reinforced with real-life examples, and practical tools are used for illustration whenever possible. An overview of the medical technology development and standards is also included in the last two chapters to provide the readers with a general concept to relate standards and regulatory control in technology development to medical technology management practice. This book is written for readers who already have a general understanding of the health care environment and are interested in getting a practical understanding of managing medical technologies. Such readers may include but are not limited to health administrators, technology planners, biomedical engineers and technologists, and supervisors and managers of technology-intensive departments. The contents are grouped into twelve chapters. Below is a brief description of each chapter:

- Chapter 1 provides an overview of technology management and introduces the systems approach to study medical technologies.

- Chapter 2 lists the benefits of managing technology using a systems approach and identifies the different phases of the technology life cycle.
- Chapter 3 discusses maintenance of medical technology including demand maintenance and preventive maintenance and the essential elements of establishing a cost-effective technology maintenance program.
- Chapter 4 describes the required infrastructure to provide effective support of medical technology. It also analyses the advantages and disadvantages of various technology support models such as in-house support, maintenance contract, self-insurance, and regional services.
- Chapter 5 outlines the importance of medical device incoming inspections and documentation and analyzes criteria for such processes. It also lists the minimum requirements of a medical equipment management database system and reviews management information that can be extracted from such database.
- Chapter 6 introduces the concept of quality improvement and covers the essential elements of a medical technology risk management program including hazard report handling, incident investigation, and training.
- Chapter 7 describes the organization, roles, and responsibilities of key stakeholders in hospital-level technology planning, assessment, prioritization, and acquisition.
- Chapter 8 introduces technology budgeting using the life cycle cost-of-ownership approach. It also discusses various financing options in technology acquisition.
- Chapter 9 leads the readers through the tendering and evaluation process in technology acquisition. It includes specification preparation, pre-purchase evaluation, and formulation of award documents.
- Chapter 10 evaluates the criteria for technology replacement and disposal of medical devices.
- Chapter 11 explores medical device standards and the standard development process. It also provides an overview of medical device regulations in the area of device risk classification and regulatory control.
- Chapter 12 gives an overview of the essential components of

design assurance and risk management in medical device development.

It is hoped that this text will enlighten readers to start using a systematic life cycle approach to manage medical technology so that appropriate technologies are used safely, effectively, and efficiently for the better of mankind.

I am indebted to my two young daughters, Victoria and Tiffany, who should have received more of my attention if I were not engaged in writing this book. I am deeply indebted to my good friend, Euclid Seeram, whose encouragement and constant reminder had made this book a reality. A number of people have contributed ideas in this book, especially Ken Yip and Stephan Bauer. I extend my special appreciation to the Biomedical Engineering Department of the Vancouver General Hospital which allowed me to include their forms and procedures in the book. Last but not the least, I want to thank Michael Thomas for agreeing, without hesitation, to publish this book upon receiving my proposal two years ago.

Anthony Y. K. Chan

CONTENTS

MEDICAL TECHNOLOGY MANAGEMENT PRACTICE

Chapter 1

INTRODUCTION TO MEDICAL TECHNOLOGY MANAGEMENT

1 OVERVIEW OF HEALTH TECHNOLOGY MANAGEMENT

Modern health care delivery and medicine are increasingly dependent on technology in the diagnosis and mitigation of illnesses, in disease prevention and in health promotion. On one hand, medical technology can be viewed as tools to improve the quality of life of individuals. On the other hand, it is considered by some as a culprit of the upward spiraling cost of health care. Nonetheless, it is one of the driving forces that shape the direction of modern health care delivery. For these reasons, it is important to manage medical technology so that it can be used appropriately, effectively, and efficiently.

Managing medical technology requires the expertise and infrastructure to address the challenges in different phases throughout the life of the technology. The "Technology Life Cycle" starts in the development phase of the technology, undergoes validation, goes through acquisition and utilization, and then terminates when it is being replaced or abandoned. This book studies the medical technology life cycle from the user's perspective, starting from technology acquisition. An overview of the development phase of medical technology at the end of the book provides the reader with a general idea of the processes involved in the design assurance, hazard analysis, and regulatory control of medical technology development.

1.1 Systems Approach to Health Technology Management

In simple terms, a system may be viewed as a group of things or parts or processes working together under certain relationships. A system transforms a set of input into a set of output entities. Within a system there are aspects, variables, or parameters which mutually act upon each other. A closed system is self-contained on a specific level and is separated from and not influenced by the environment, whereas an open system is influenced by the environmental conditions by which it is surrounded. Figure 1–1 shows an example of a system. The elements within the system and their relationships as well as the environment can affect the performance of the system. A more complicated system may contain multiple numbers of subsystems or simple systems.

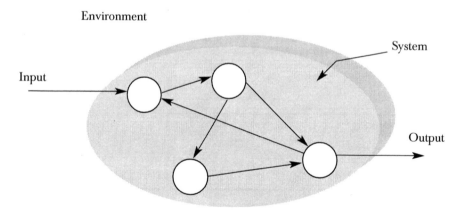

Figure 1–1. Example of a System.

In analyzing a large complex system, one can break down the system into several smaller subsystems with the output from one subsystem connected to the input of another. A basic subsystem comprises of input, output, and processes as shown in Figure 1–2. The process that takes the output and feed it back into the input in order to modify the output is called a feedback process. A system with feedback is called a closed loop system, whereas a system without any feedback is called an open loop system. Most systems that we encounter contain feedback paths and hence are closed loop systems.

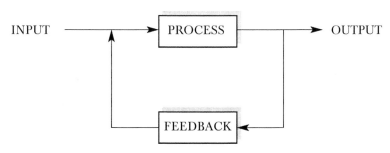

Figure 1–2. A Closed Loop System.

Listening to a radio is an example of a simple closed loop system. The input to the system is the broadcast in the form of electromagnetic wave that is received by the radio. The radio processes the received signal and produces the audible sound such as music. If the music (the output) is not loud enough, the listener will turn up the volume to increase the sound level. In doing so, the listener becomes the feedback process that analyzes the loudness of the music and produces the action to turn up the volume.

Figure 1–3a shows the block diagram of an asynchronous (fixed rate) pacemaker. The pulse generator produces a pulse at a predetermined rate (e.g. 60 pulses per minute). These pulses are transmitted to the ventricle of the heart via a lead wire and an electrode to stimulate the ventricle to contract. Pulses are sent to the heart irrespective of the natural heart activities. Figure 1–3b shows a demand pacemaker. In addition to the pulse generator, the lead, and electrode, the natural contraction signal from the heart is sensed and transmitted back to the pacemaker. With the feedback, the pacemaker is able to skip sending stimulation to the heart if it is detected to be beating on its own. The fixed rate pacemaker in this example is an open loop system, whereas the demand pacemaker is a closed loop system.

A systems approach is a generalized technique to understand organized complexity. It provides a unified framework and instigates a way

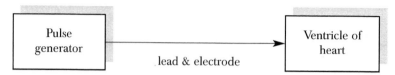

Figure 1–3a. Fixed Rate Pacemaker–an Open Loop System.

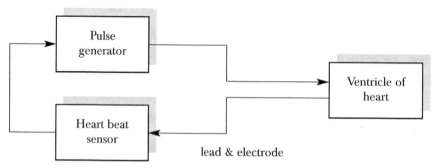

Figure 1–3b. Demand Pacemaker–a Closed Loop System.

of thinking about all the entities and their relationships. A systems approach can be used to solve problems within a complex environment. By looking at all components within the system and analyzing the input and output of each subsystem, one can isolate the problem and establish the relationships of the problem with respect to each component in the system.

For example, cellular phone technology is used in telecommunication. A cellular communication system includes the users (yourself and whomever you want to talk to), a service provider (e.g., AT&T), some equipment (cell phones, transmitters, switches, etc.), and the transmission medium (electromagnetic wave in the atmosphere). These components within the system all work together and each plays a role to achieve the objective, that is, to convey the information in real time with minimal distortion from one user to another. A weak link in any part of the system will degrade the quality of the system. For example, one may experience poor reception when making a phone call inside an elevator. In this case, the user is in a sub-optimal transmission medium for the communication system to operate effectively.

Similarly, a sub-optimal component (e.g., inadequate staff training after a new technology is deployed) in health care may decrease the overall efficacy and increase the risk on patients under care. In order to achieve the desired objectives, one should adopt a systems approach to manage technology in the healthcare environment.

Health care is an extremely complex system, medical technology is a subsystem of the health care system and is by itself very complicated. A study of health technology management requires a good understanding of the sub-subsystems within this complicated subsystem. In addition, one needs to understand the distinct perspectives of the different hierarchical levels. For example, perspectives of government policy makers are different from those of hospital department managers.

2 HEALTH TECHNOLOGY MANAGEMENT PROGRAM

2.1 Elements of a Health Technology Management Program

Health technology in the broad sense includes devices, supplies, drugs, medical techniques, and procedures used in the monitoring, diagnosis, and treatment of patients as well as in disease prevention and health improvement. Figure 1–4 shows the main elements of a technology management program. This book focuses on management of health technology in hospital settings, in specific, on management of medical device and supply technologies. Nevertheless, these concepts can readily be extended to other aspects of health technology. To differentiate it from the bigger picture of health technology management, we adopt the definition by Yadin David and Thomas Jude[1] who

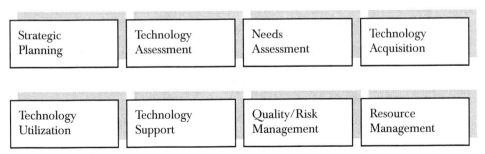

Figure 1–4. Elements of a Technology Management Program.

1. David, Yadin and Jude, Thomas M. *Medical Technology Management, Biomedical Measurement Series,* Spacelabs Medical, Inc., 1993.

stated, "Medical Technology Management is an interdisciplinary program that utilizes acceptable methods and information to provide guidelines and qualifications for the planning, selection, procurement, utilization, maintenance, and replacement of medical hardware, software and supplies."

2.2 Key Stakeholders in Medical Technology Management

In order to manage medical technology properly, one needs to first identify the stakeholders involved in the deployment and use of medical technology in the healthcare system. Listed below are the key stakeholders of medical technology management in a hospital setting. It should be obvious that in most cases, clinical areas that treat patients are the end users of medical technology.

- Technology users in clinical areas.
- Biomedical or clinical engineering is responsible for the initial evaluation and ongoing support of medical technology.
- Physical Plant provides a suitable environment for its operation.
- The Purchasing Department is responsible for acquisition, tracking, and disposal of medical technology.
- The Central Supplies Department ensures the cleanliness and sterility of the devices as well as providing the users with operational supplies and consumables.
- Information Services takes care of the computing and data communication needs of the technology.

These allied health professionals form an intricate system and each serves an important role to ensure the availability and reliability of the technology. In a health care facility, a number of committees are involved in various aspects of technology management such as technology deployment and risk and quality assurance. Some of the more common technology management committees are listed below:

- The Medical Technology Advisory Committee (MTAC)
- The Capital Budget Committee (CBC)
- The Product Standards Committee (PSC)

The MTAC focuses on the strategic planning and assessment of medical technology. The CBC focuses on the needs analysis, capital equipment prioritization, and acquisition. The PSC ensures that technology under consideration complies with current standards of practice and is compatible with existing components and processes in the facility. The above-mentioned key stakeholders and senior administrative staff members of the health facility are usually standing members of these committees. The roles and functions of these committees are discussed in later chapters.

Chapter 2

MEDICAL TECHNOLOGY LIFE CYCLE

1 A SYSTEMS APPROACH TO TECHNOLOGY MANAGEMENT

A systematic way to evaluate a medical technology is to analyze the various phases of the technology from its acquisition to disposal. A systems approach to technology management will assist the health facility in realizing the following benefits:

- optimize the technology assessment and acquisition processes
- reduce costs in technology acquisition, operation, and maintenance
- increase utilization, efficiency, and reliability of the technology
- improve quality of care through appropriate deployment of technology and use of quality assurance measures
- reduce hazards through effective technology risk management

One can use the example of a motor vehicle ownership to illustrate the concepts of technology management. Consider the following process:

1. A person who is considering to purchase a vehicle has to consider the needs of owning a vehicle. Is this vehicle for pleasure or for business? What is the seating capacity? Is comfort more

important than economy?

2. After he or she has decided on the vehicle type, the next step will be comparing prices of different makes and price shopping at different dealerships.

3. Test driving to get a real feeling of the vehicle is often a critical step in the acquisition process.

4. A decision on a particular make and model is made.

5. With some negotiation, a purchase agreement is signed specifying the details of the purchase.

6. Upon delivery, the sales person explains to the new owner the features and operation of the vehicle. After finished checking everything is in order, the owner signs an acceptance document. The owner then drives the vehicle home and shows it to his or her family.

7. During the lifetime of the vehicle, the owner needs to take it to scheduled maintenance (e.g., 180,000 km service) and take care of the odd breakdowns and repairs.

8. A common question a vehicle owner has to face is whether the maintenance and repair is done at the dealer's service department or at the cheaper street corner repair shop.

9. The cost of maintaining the vehicle includes insurance, gas, maintenance, etc. (and of course, traffic violation tickets).

10. The owner may receive recall notices from the manufacturer. Recalls can be minor (such as problem with a light switch) or life threatening (such as potential fuel line leaks).

11. After years of usage, the owner may consider replacing the vehicle. The urge of replacement may be due to declining reliability (e.g., it broke down on the highway twice in the last month) or changing needs (e.g., a passenger van is needed due to starting a family).

12. Before shopping for a new one, the owner has to decide whether to trade-in the old vehicle at the dealership or list it in the "Buy and Sell" newspaper.

13. The above will repeat itself as long as our vehicle owner continues to own a vehicle.

2 THE MEDICAL TECHNOLOGY LIFE CYCLE

A systematic way to manage medical technology is to study and optimize all phases in the useful life of the medical technology, or study and optimize the technology life cycle. The technology life cycle of a medical device from the user's perspective is shown in Figure 2–1. It starts at the planning and acquisition phase, through the acceptance process, being used in the clinical environment, and then eventually being replaced after it has reached the end of its useful life. The acquisition, acceptance, and replacement of a technology happen only once in the life of the technology; however, technology utilization involves a number of activities and each can occur multiple times. We can therefore further break down this medical technology life cycle into two sub-cycles, namely, the acquisition and utilization sub-cycles (Fig. 2–2).

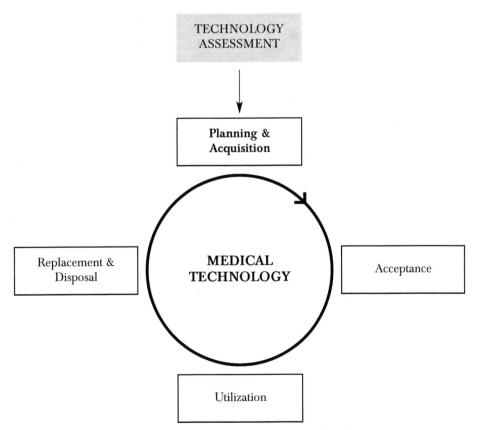

Figure 2–1. Medical Technology Life Cycle.

2.1 Acquisition Sub-cycle

The acquisition sub-cycle includes the following phases:
• Technology Assessment
• Technology Planning
• Acquisition
• Acceptance
• Replacement and Disposal

In this sub-cycle, a technology will go through each of the above phases once and will eventually be replaced by a new technology.

2.2 Utilization Sub-cycle

The utilization sub-cycle includes the following phases:
• Training
• Maintenance
• Quality Assurance
• Risk Management

A technology can go through this sub-cycle as many times as it is necessary until it is retired or replaced. The decision to remove the technology is often made in the acquisition sub-cycle, but it is influenced by the outcomes of the utilization sub-cycle.

In fact, this life cycle approach of medical technology management can be applied to any technology. The vehicle ownership example discussed earlier can be analyzed using the life-cycle approach. Table 2–1 shows the different phases of this life cycle. We will examine in details these phases in the remainder of this book.

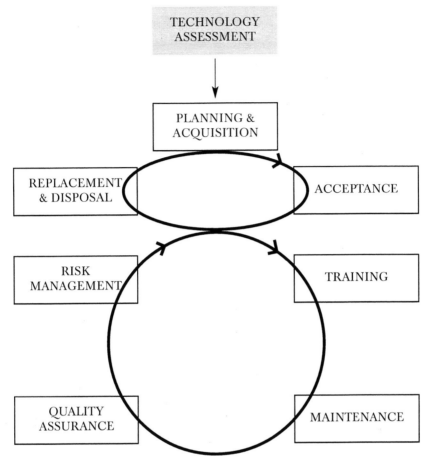

Figure 2–2. Medical Technology Life Cycle.

Table 2–1

EXAMPLE OF LIFE-CYCLE APPROACH IN TECHNOLOGY MANAGEMENT

Phase of Life Cycle	Decisions to make when owning a motor vehicle
Assessment	What type of vehicle do I need? How many seats? An all wheel drive?
Planning	Can I afford it? Do I have parking at work?
Acquisition	Negotiation with dealer. Price shopping. Sign under the dotted line.
Acceptance	Should I bring the vehicle home and make an appointment afterwards to fix the small scratch on the hood?
Replacement & Disposal	Is my old car still worth something? Trade-in?
Utilization	Do I sign up for car-pooling? Should I use regular or premium gas?
Training	Should I teach my 16-year-old to drive? Or send her to a driving school?
Maintenance	My car needs a tune-up. Does this cheaper street corner garage do as good a job as the dealer?
Quality Assurance	Should I adhere to the maintenance and inspection schedule?
Risk Management	I received a tire defect recall but I need the vehicle for a vacation trip tomorrow. Should I postpone my vacation or rent a vehicle or ignore the recall until after the trip?

Chapter 3

TECHNOLOGY MAINTENANCE

Demand maintenance (DM), sometimes called unscheduled maintenance, includes works initiated from device failure and modifications. Whereas scheduled maintenance refers to device preventative maintenance (PM) and performance verification. This chapter covers the fundamentals of establishing a medical device demand and preventive maintenance program in a healthcare facility.

1 DEMAND MAINTENANCE

Many of the in-house medical technology management programs in existence today began with the need to repair basic medical devices found in hospitals. These programs were usually attached to the existing in-house maintenance programs under the physical plant departments. As medical devices became more complex, and especially with the introduction of electrical-operated medical devices, the need for skilled workforce to support such specialized technologies has drastically increased. Of significant interest was the interaction of electricity with patients, which therefore created the notion to prevent accidental electrocution. In conjunction with the many documented cases of patient injuries when flammable anesthetic gases were ignited by electrical-operated equipment, many healthcare facilities started to employ specially trained personnel to support and manage their in-house medical technology, thereby creating the in-house medical technology management department–the Biomedical or Clinical Engineering Department.

It may perhaps be stated that the "bread and butter" of many technology management programs, and the foundation of an in-house clinical engineering department, is the repair or corrective maintenance (CM) of medical devices in the facility. Medical devices produced today are designed to minimize electrical shock hazard to both patients and clinical staff. Anesthetic gases in use today are, by law, no longer highly flammable. Although medical devices still suffer from occasional failures, incidents that are related to the above mentioned causes have been drastically reduced. Generally speaking, all medical device malfunctions may be classified under one of the following three headings:

1. Malfunctions caused by medical device failure
2. Problems caused by misuse (usually due to inadequate or improper user education)
3. Unusual physiological or multiple-device interaction that may cause problems or confusions to medical and support staff

1.1 Elements of Cost-Effective Demand Maintenance

Device malfunctions are rectified through systematic troubleshooting (that is, isolation of the problem using systems approach). This is done by trained technologists with a combination of education and experience. This combination of knowledge includes the symptoms of problems, the principles of medical device operation and their interaction with the patients, and basic anatomy and physiology as well as engineering knowledge. The repair (i.e., the replacement or correction of components or subsystems in order to restore the device to its normal operating state) may consist of replacing an entire module or actually troubleshooting and repairing down to the component level. The actual repair performed, often somewhere between these

two extremes, is dependent upon a number of factors including:
- the complexity of the device
- the knowledge of the technologist
- the tolerable downtime
- the availability of service information
- the availability of replacement parts
- the cost of repair including labor and parts

Cost–effective repair of medical devices requires thorough understanding of the problems and the constraints. A common problem preventing cost-effective repair of medical devices is the lack of technical information to in-house service personnel. Technical information is usually contained in the device service manual available from the device manufacturer. Oftentimes, a purchasing staff is not aware of the importance of such information. As a result, service manuals were either not purchased or not specified in the purchase order. Most manufacturers would provide service manuals free to equipment buyers if they were specified in the purchase agreement. However, the quality and the amount of information contained in the manuals may vary substantially from one manufacturer to another. Therefore, health care facilities should specify and evaluate the service documentation in their device acquisition processes. At the minimum, a comprehensive service manual should contain:
- device specifications
- a description of the operation and precautions
- a functional building block diagram
- a detailed theory of operation including technical description of functional blocks and signal flow between modules and components
- performance verification procedures
- a trouble shooting guide
- a component layout diagram
- a wiring diagram
- a full schematic diagram, and
- a parts list

In summary, the successfulness of an in-house repair service is dependent upon:
- competent service personnel
- availability of proper test equipment and tools
- availability of technical information, i.e., comprehensive service

manuals
- readily accessible and reasonably priced replacement parts
- cooperation of user departments
- support from Administration (e.g., resource allocations)

1.2 Problem Recording

There is a definite need to track problems associated with a particular device. Users should be encouraged to identify the symptoms of the problem and record them in the service request. The user reporting the problem should complete a service requisition with the following information and send it alongside with the defective device:
- a description and identification of the device to be serviced
- a summary of the symptoms of the problem
- identity of the person reporting the problem
- date and time of the service request
- location of the device, contact person, phone number

The technologist who performed the service should complete the remaining information.
- a description of the repair action (include what is done to rectify the problem, components repaired or replaced, performance verification results after repair, etc.)
- a list of replacement parts or components used
- time taken to perform the service
- identity of the person who performed the service
- date and time of service completion

Examples of a "Service Requisition" and a "Service Report" are shown in Figures 3–1a and b.

Medical Equipment Service Requisition				
Clinical Area:		Requested By:		Signature:
Priority: Normal - ❏ High - ❏		Date:		Local:
Device Type:			Device ID:	
Detailed Description of Problem:				
Please attach completed form to the device to be serviced				

Figure 3–1a. Equipment Service Requisition Form.

**BIOMEDICAL ENGINEERING
SERVICE REPORT**

SERVICE TYPE		COMPLAINT			PROBLEM		
Preventive Maintenance	☐	Adjustment	☐	1	Inservice	☐	1
Demand Maintenance	☐	Alarms	☐	2	Research	☐	2
Other Productive Work	☐	Broken	☐	3	Calibrate/Adjust	☐	3
Incoming Inspection	☐	Interference	☐	4	Peripherals	☐	4
		Noisy	☐	5	Electrical	☐	5
Equipment ID# _____		Non-functional	☐	6	Mechanical	☐	6
Description _____		Output	☐	7	Operator	☐	7
		Parts Missing	☐	8	Comments	☐	8
Technologist _____		PM-Generated	☐	9	Upgrade	☐	9
Repair Hours _____		No Information	☐	0	None	☐	0
Date Completed YY_____MM_____DD_____							

Day	Hours	Comments and/or Corrective Action

Part #	Parts Description	Qty.	Price Ea.	Subtotal
	SHOP MATERIALS			
			TOTAL	

ELECTRICAL SAFETY TESTS

☐ Battery Operated

Grounding Resistance (Ω)			Current When Ground Open (μA)						Current Through Ground (μA)		
Case			Power Switch	Line Normal		Line Reverse			Power Switch	Line Normal	Line Reverse
				Case	Other	Case	Other				
Other			Off						Off		
			On						On		

Figure 3–1b. Equipment Service Report Form.

2 PREVENTIVE MAINTENANCE

Preventive maintenance includes visual inspection, functional verification, calibration, cleaning, lubrication, and replacement of components that may wear out or fail. The intention is to identify existing problems and to prevent foreseeable failures.

There are many terms used to describe the maintenance of medical devices (or any equipment, for that matter). Below are some common interpretations:

Maintenance–The function of keeping devices in a safe, functional and calibrated state through the use of a variety of both corrective and preventive maintenance functions. All of the following functions are covered by the general term of maintenance.

Performance Verification (also known as *Functional Testing, Quality Assurance Inspection,* or *Performance Assurance Inspection*)–To confirm that the device is operable, and that the accuracy of the equipment's function and measure is within established and reasonable guidelines. This may be performed by the operator in the area where the device is used or by a trained technologist in a laboratory. Performance verification is done through a comparison of the device to a reference standard, usually traceable to a primary standard.

Calibration–To rectify, through adjustment or repair, any discrepancy between a device's output or performance as indicated by the difference between a device measurement and some reference standard. Oftentimes calibration requires specialized tools and complicated procedures and is therefore best left to a trained person such as a biomedical engineering technologist.

While the importance of operator performance verification is not to be underemphasized, this section will concentrate primarily on the issue of preventive maintenance performed by trained service personnel such as biomedical engineering technologists.

2.1 The Importance of Performing Preventive Maintenance

The purpose of performing periodic inspection, preventive maintenance (PM), and quality assurance (QA) inspections is five-fold.

1. *Reducing the risk of injury*–Preventive maintenance assists in minimizing the risk of injury to patients, staff, and others in the healthcare facility.
2. *Regulatory compliance*–To maintain its accreditation, healthcare facilities must prove that equipment used in the facility complies with all relevant codes, standards, and regulations. In the

absence of these, the facility must prove that the maintenance recommendations of equipment manufacturers are reasonably followed.

3. *Performance assurance*–By scheduling maintenance at an appropriate interval, minor operational problems can be discovered and corrected in order to ensure accurate diagnostic or therapeutic results.

4. *Minimizing downtime*–Scheduled preventive maintenance helps to ensure that the facility gets its maximum use of the equipment by minimizing the need for unscheduled maintenance which often results in the need to reschedule or cancel procedures. In the case of critical technology, such as expensive diagnostic imaging equipment, failure will lead to procedure cancellation and revenue loss.

5. *Avoiding excessive repair*–While unscheduled maintenance is almost always a reality of any piece of equipment, scheduled preventive maintenance will assist in reducing the potential for large, excessive repair expenses.

2.2 Establishing Inclusion Guidelines

A typical acute care hospital has a few thousand pieces of medical equipment in its inventory; some are highly complex devices such as a catheterization laboratory monitoring system while others can be as simple as a liquid-filled thermometer. Ideally, these devices should all be inspected periodically. However, in practice, in order to put resources into better use, not all devices are included into a preventive maintenance program. PM can be performed in-house, under warranty, by the manufacturer, or by a third-party organization. Oftentimes the identification of which equipment should be placed on a preventive maintenance schedule is based solely on the recommendation of the manufacturer, or on the recommendation of qualified in-house personnel. Listed below are two suggested guidelines for devices to be included in a preventive maintenance program:

- Electromedical devices including all diagnostic and therapeutic equipment that have contact with the patient both directly, such as using catheters or electrodes, and indirectly, such as those using electromagnetic radiation or ultrasound.
- Devices whose accuracy and performance have a direct impact

on the health outcome of patients and the deterioration of device performance may not be obvious to its users.

Other than special devices used in healthcare, many commercially available devices may become hazardous when used in the health-care environment. For example, television sets and other recreational electronics, while under normal use are safe by themselves, may create an electrocution hazard when combined with medical equipment (e.g., an implanted metal lead wire can conduct a very small yet fatal current from a table fan to the patient's heart). It is very common that patients insist on bringing their own personal electronic devices to the bedside. Under these circumstances, facilities are wise to consult technical experts who can assist in establishing reasonable and executable policies to deal with these problems.

In any case, regardless of whether or not the device is placed on scheduled maintenance, many regulatory bodies require that maintenance decision to be documented before the device is put into use. The documentation of a medical device's scheduled maintenance decision must include both the equipment inspection frequency and the maintenance procedure.

2.3 Frequency of Inspection

Establishing the frequency of preventative maintenance is quite difficult due to the fact that many factors impact on a particular device's requirement for maintenance: usage, operational procedures, device age, etc. For a single device, e.g., a cardiac defibrillator, a weekly inspection in a coronary care hospital may be required and substantiated. However, the same device in a general hospital may only need a maintenance check every three to six months. The same could be true regarding who should perform the inspection of the device. For example, some hospitals have daily rounds made by biomedical engineering technologists to perform functional checks and inspect filters and hoses on anesthetic machines, others may have the same work done by respiratory therapists, and still others require the anesthetists to perform the same inspection. Tied in with the frequency of the inspection is the nature of inspection. In the two examples described above, the inspection is not necessarily preventive maintenance inspection, but mainly operational performance verification.

One of the most popular methods of establishing the inspection frequency is adhering to the very strict recommendations of the device manufacturer. This could be one of the preferred methods, since manufacturers are most aware of the device requirements and should also be aware of the environmental impact of their devices. However, the manufacturer's recommended inspection schedules are often biased toward an excessive number of maintenance procedures as well as too frequent parts replacements. Such high inspection frequency is to ensure that the device is always within specifications even operating under the worst case scenario. Inspections that are too frequent are not cost effective and provide little return, especially when PMs require expensive replacement parts, such as filters, hoses, chemicals, etc. In some cases, it may even reduce the expected life span of the device. On the other extreme, if the inspection is insufficient, it may adversely affect the accuracy and reliability of the device and even patient safety.

Due to the above-mentioned factors, a hospital should have qualified personnel to establish appropriate inspection frequencies. These frequencies should be based on the manufacturer's recommended schedules, knowledge of the equipment, the clinical environment, and the equipment service histories. As a starting point, one can refer to the recommendations and guidelines published by organizations such as ECRI (a non-profit consumer council of medical technologies in U.S. URL: http://www.ecri.org) or the local regulatory authority such as the CSA in Canada (Canadian Standards Association. URL: http://www.csa.com).

To maintain a cost-effective PM program, especially when the in-house service department is facing limited resources and a big workload, it is necessary to establish a reasonable inspection frequency for the device as well as a priority system to prioritize preventive maintenance inspections. When establishing the priority for PM, a number of well-documented factors must be taken into consideration. Such factors include:
- risk associated with using the device
- clinical application
- availability of spare or loaner equipment
- device failure rate
- maintenance requirements
- manufacturer's recommendations
- revenue lost due to downtime

- available resources for PM inspection
- cost of service

For example, a piece of life supporting equipment whose misuse or failure could cause serious harm will need to be inspected more frequently than equipment that has a lower associated risk. A device whose unavailability could cause cancellation of procedures may need to be inspected more often. To establish PM priorities, each device should be assessed and ranked using a set of criteria. Examples of such criteria include:

- physical risk
- functional requirements
- maintenance requirements

An example of establishing a PM priority system for medical device is as follows:

In this ranking system, medical devices are assigned a score in each of the 4 categories: patient and operator safety, performance, availability, and demand for service.

Patient and operator safety: Will injury result from the machine malfunction?
- No, the machine will not likely to be dangerous–0
- Yes, however, the malfunction should be detected by the operator–6
- Yes, it is unlikely that the malfunction will be detected by the operator–12

Performance: Will the quality of care be adversely affected by the malfunction?
- No–0
- Yes, however, the malfunction should be detected by the operator–4
- Yes, it is unlikely that the malfunction will be detected by the operator–8

Availability: How important is it that the equipment is available?
- A backup unit is always available; downtime is not critical–0
- An alternative method of providing patient care may be arranged–3
- No backup or substitution is available; the equipment is vital to patient care–6

Demand for service: How often does the machine need to be serviced to keep it functional and up to standards?
- Seldom–0
- Average–2
- Frequently–4

The PM priority number is the sum of all the scores for the device. All devices are ranked and their PM priority numbers computed accordingly. For example, a cardiac defibrillator may have a score of 12, 8, 6 & 2 in the above categories. Hence, the PM priority number is 28. The higher the number, the higher is the PM priority. A time factor is also built into the system to escalate the equipment priority if it has passed its scheduled inspection date. In this scheme, the PM priority is multiplied by one plus the number of scheduled inspections it has missed. For example, if a device has a PM priority of 20 and has missed one inspection, the adjusted priority will be 20 x 2 = 40.

The PM priority is computed automatically by a computer program and printed out in the PM work scheduled. In this way, the technologists may start to perform PM inspections according to the priority assigned.

2.4 PM Inspection Procedures

Closely associated with the frequency of inspection is the need to specify what maintenance is to be performed on a device, that is, specific maintenance procedures need to be developed and documented for each device and each type of inspection. This will ensure that maintenance work is done consistently without omissions and will not vary from person to person. What is inspected is dependent on the equipment being serviced. Inspection procedures are to be written for each device type, or preferably, for each unique model of medical device. For example, defibrillators from two different manufacturers will each have their own PM schedule and inspection checklist. These procedures need to be periodically reviewed and revised as required. Associated with the procedures are the forms used to document the test results. Many service departments have moved away from the traditional "paper-intensive office" and have gone to recording test results directly into a computerized equipment database. Documentation requirements for medical technology maintenance will be discussed in more detail in another chapter.

An example of a PM inspection form of an ECG monitor is shown in Figure 3–2. The inspection form documents the device's identification, the date and time of the PM, who did the work, and what was done, including the results of tests performed and the acceptable tolerances if applicable. Note that only the names of the tests are listed in the inspection form. The actual procedures and instructions of the tests are to be documented as well.

IPM Form for ECG Monitors (Major)
Hospital – Biomedical Engineering

Work Order No.: _____ Location: _____ Control No.: _____
Manufacturer: _____ Model: _____ Serial: _____

──────────── TEST APPARATUS REQUIRED ────────────

[ ] Leakage Current Meter/Safety Analy   [ ] ECG Simulator, Variable Output/Rate
[ ] Ground Resistance Ohmmeter

──────────── SUPPLIES REQUIRED ────────────

[ ] Ruler, Metric, Transparent

──────────── QUALITATIVE TASKS ────────────

[ ] Chassis/Housing   [ ] Controls/Switches
[ ] Mount   [ ] Battery/Charger
[ ] Casters/Brakes   [ ] Indicators/Displays
[ ] AC Plug/Receptacle   [ ] CRT Display
[ ] Line Cord   [ ] 1 mV Step Response
[ ] Strain Reliefs   [ ] Alarms
[ ] Circuit Breaker/Fuse   [ ] Audible Signals
[ ] Cables   [ ] Labeling
[ ] Connectors   [ ] Direct Writer
[ ] Electrodes

──────────── PREVENTIVE MAINTENANCE TASKS ────────────

[ ] Clean Exterior and Accessories   [ ] Replace Filters and Batteries
[ ] Lubricate Chart Recorder

──────────── QUANTITATIVE TASKS ────────────

Task Description/Criterion	Set	Indicd	Measured	Pass	Fail
Grounding Resistance $\leq 0.5\ \Omega$			_____	[ ]	[ ]
Chassis Leakage Current $\leq 100\ \mu A$			_____	[ ]	[ ]
Rate Calibration $\pm 5\%$ or 5 bpm at 60 and 120 bpm	___	___	___	[ ] [ ]	[ ] [ ]
Rate Alarm $\pm 5\%$ or 5bpm at 40 and 120 bpm	___	___	___	[ ] [ ]	[ ] [ ]

──────────── SUMMARY ────────────

NOTES:

[ ] Service Required   [ ] Removed from Use   [ ] Acceptable for Use

Completed by	Date	IPM Time	Repair Time

Figure 3–2. PM Inspection Form of ECG Monitor.

Chapter 4

ORGANIZATION OF SUPPORT SERVICES

A well-organized, medical technology management program is critical to the safe and cost-effective use of medical technology in a healthcare facility. Medical technology support may be obtained from in-house personnel or external contractors. A hospital may acquire medical technology support service through a variety of service arrangements. This chapter discusses the infrastructure and key criteria to establish a medical technology maintenance program.

1 CENTRALIZED VERSUS DECENTRALIZED MODEL

Servicing medical devices in a facility can be centralized or distributed. In a distributed model, the responsibility to maintain medical devices lies with the device users. In contrast, all maintaining activities are coordinated by a single department in a centralized model (e.g., the Biomedical Engineering Department). In general, a centralized medical technology maintenance arrangement is preferred.

1.1 Benefits of a Centralized Equipment Service Arrangement

Many hospitals and healthcare facilities, which lack a centralized medical technology maintenance program, are at a great disadvantage when it comes to cost-effectiveness in equipment support and maintenance.

A typical healthcare facility with a decentralized maintenance system has some of its devices under warranty service, some maintained by in-house personnel, and some maintained by outside service vendors (under service agreements). Maintenance requests are initiated and monitored by the individual user departments. When a device is in need of maintenance (e.g., repair), the user must first determine whom to contact to perform the work. The user will have to keep track of the progress to ensure that the equipment is serviced promptly and correctly as well as to verify the completion of work and the associated documentation. Time will be taken away from the normal duty of the individual who performed the above functions.

Under a centralized medical technology maintenance arrangement, all equipment services, whether performed by in-house staff or by external contractors, are managed by one department. User departments only need to phone one location to report problems and are no longer concerned with the monitoring and documentation of the maintenance work. With this arrangement, departments are be relieved of the responsibility of equipment maintenance, allowing their staff to carry out their assigned duties and thereby improving departmental efficiency.

Furthermore, without appropriate technical knowledge, most users are unable to assess the services rendered by the external service providers nor able to determine the appropriate level of service required for their equipment. This situation may lead to expensive service costs, unnecessary equipment repair, and premature equipment replacement.

When each department independently solicits its own equipment service, it is difficult or impossible to negotiate with outside service vendors. Under a centralized arrangement, based on the economy of scale, a hospital can negotiate with service vendors and usually be able to achieve savings on equipment service contracts.

1.2 Comprehensive Maintenance and Support Service

The overall goal of a comprehensive maintenance and support service is to ensure that all equipment within the healthcare facility is properly maintained to a satisfactory level of safety and performance, while at the same time ensuring that it is accomplished in the most efficient, responsible, and controlled manner possible. Under such an arrangement, in addition to coordinating all medical technology maintenance activities, the central department also employs technical staff to perform a substantial amount of the maintenance work. The support and repair of equipment has been and continues to be the primary responsibility of the Biomedical Engineering Department (BMED) in many hospitals. These departments have repeatedly demonstrated cost-effectiveness and immense benefits in medical technology support and maintenance.

2 SERVICE MODALITIES

In this section, the various means of servicing medical equipment are discussed, along with their relative advantages and disadvantages. Commonly used service modalities include:
- in-house service
- contracted service
- maintenance insurance
- contracted technology management

Depending on the circumstances and resources available, an

appropriate mix of different modalities will result in the best cost-effective solution for maintaining and managing medical technology in the facility.

2.1 In-House Service

2.1.1 Factors Affecting the Effectiveness of In-house Service

In-house service refers to maintaining the equipment by employees of the healthcare facility. The technologists and engineers in the Biomedical Engineering Department (BMED) often provide such services on medical technology. The Hospital Information System Department (HISD) looks after computer needs. Physical Plant Services (PPS) looks after the "hotel" services of the facility. In regards to medical technology, PPS may be responsible for the central medical gas supply system, nurse call system, wheelchairs, patient beds, etc. The primary responsibility of the Central Supplies Department (CSD) is the distribution of medical supplies and disinfection/sterilization of medical devices. In some hospitals, CSD is responsible to dispatch, clean, and provide first level maintenance on simple and high-volume devices such as electronic thermometers and infusion pumps. Depending on historical factors and the expertise available in the various departments, the boundaries between these hospital departments are often quite fuzzy.

Many hospitals have achieved substantial cost saving by eliminating external service contracts and assuming the service responsibilities by in-house personnel. This successfulness of in-house service is dependent on a list of factors that must be examined before such a decision is made. Some of these factors are listed below:
- the cost of the service contract
- the number of preventive maintenance (PM) and estimated repair requests for the equipment
- the work hours and staffing costs associated with the PM and repair
- availability of technical information and replacement parts
- hardware and software replacement costs
- availability of special test equipment and tools including diagnostic software
- the level of expertise available to perform the work

• the acceptable downtime of the equipment

By assessing these factors in the equipment acquisition phase and thereafter periodically, the hospital's centralized service provider (e.g., BMED) can evaluate whether or not in-house personnel can, in a cost-effective manner, assume the service responsibility of the medical technology. Based on the outcome of the analysis, in-house service may completely avoid a service contract or perform partial servicing and repair in order to reduce the overall maintenance cost. As the in-house service program develops and acquires more experience, it may be possible to expand the maintenance responsibility, thereby reducing maintenance costs while maintaining or even improving the level of service to the equipment users.

On a periodic basis, meetings should be held between equipment user departments and the centralized service provider to review the statistics of equipment service, including equipment covered under service contracts and those serviced by in-house personnel.

2.1.2 Budgeting Strategies

There are two common methods to finance equipment maintenance in a hospital or other healthcare facility. Both of these systems have their respective advantages and disadvantages.

1. The first method is to assign a central maintenance and repair budget to the centralized service provider (CSP). The CSP would have full control of the budget and be responsible for all maintaining activities. Under this arrangement, the CSP has full discretion to assign maintenance service to its in-house personnel or external service providers.

2. The second method to finance maintenance is through a charge-back system. Under this arrangement, the maintenance budget is distributed among the user departments. The CSP cross charges the user department for the maintenance service performed. The users in general have more influence in the service activities as they are paying for the services performed.

The main advantage of centralizing repair budgets is the added control and flexibility to the CSP under such an arrangement. As demand maintenance is often unpredictable, the CSP could use financial surpluses in certain departments to even out shortages in others. Also, surpluses could be used to buy frequently used spare parts for future use. The major disadvantage of a centralized budgeting is the fact that user departments are no longer fiscally responsible for the equipment and thus may not put as much effort to prevent accident and abuse of equipment. A second possible disadvantage is the fact that user departments no longer know how much it costs to maintain certain equipment, and therefore do not know the overall cost of the programs they are offering. However, these shortcomings may be overcome through some administrative measures.

The charge-back system has the advantage that users are fiscally responsible for ensuring that the equipment is properly cared-for, while at the same time giving them a better idea about the cost of maintenance of the equipment. This system, however, has a disadvantage that it may lead to underservicing as departments may, in order to save money for other uses, only ask for repair work and ignore preventive maintenance. Underservicing will increase equipment-related risks and degrade quality of care. However, by establishing a minimum service level (i.e., PM frequencies and procedures) for the equipment at the time of device purchase, this problem can be prevented. Other disadvantages of the charge-back system include the increased complexity of record keeping and paperwork, plus the loss of control by the CSP over individual departments' maintenance budgets which could result in the loss of overall hospital savings.

In either method, it is important to track the costs of both in-house and external maintenance services. This information is vital in order to determine the best combination of service modalities and can be used in considering technology replacement and acquisition.

2.1.3 Requirements for Establishing an In-house Service Department

HUMAN RESOURCES REQUIREMENTS. The first step to establish an in-house service program is to estimate the required number and mix of in-house service personnel. One approach is based on the assumption that the number of acute care beds in a hospital correlates with the amount of technology present, which in turn correlates to the number of staff required to service the technology. There are some published statistics and guidelines on the staffing level per acute care bed (e.g., the Clinical Engineering Manual, Scientific Enterprises Inc., 1988). Another approach is to estimate the staffing requirements based on the time required to perform the medical equipment services.

The second approach, which takes into account the device inventory being supported and the level of services required, provides a more realistic estimate of the staffing requirements. To obtain a realistic estimate, this method requires detailed information about the medical device inventory, PM frequency and time, estimated failure rate and repair time, productivity patterns, and a hospital's policies and procedures on medical equipment services. Based upon these data, the total service time and hence the number of full-time equivalent (FTE) of support staff can be calculated. While this method may only be an estimate, it does provide a starting point from which the actual FTE can be adjusted when the actual workload statistics are available. An example to estimate PM FTE is shown below:

A community hospital is planning to establish an in-house medical equipment service program. In order to calculate the FTE needed to perform PM services for the medical equipment, the following estimates of PM frequency and PM time are used:

Device Type	Number of Devices	PM Freq. (no./yr)	PM Time (hr/PM)	Calculated PM Time (hr/yr)
A	500	1	1	500
B	400	2	2	1,600
C	50	4	1.5	300
			Total hrs	2,400

The above calculation shows that a total of 2,400 hours of PM time is needed. If the working hours of one full-time biomedical engineering technologist is 2,000 hours per year and assuming the productivity is 70%, the time devoted to actual PM work is 2,000 x 0.70 = 1,400 hours per year. Therefore, the number of FTE needed to perform the PM is equal to 2,400/1,400 = 1.7 FTE.

OTHER REQUIREMENTS. In addition to human resources, the following requirements need to be considered when establishing an in-house service department.
   • Workshop–The workshop should have enough physical space to perform the necessary work, to hold equipment waiting for

repair or pick up, to store spare parts, and to file service documentation. Ideally, the in-house service department should be close to and have easy access to service-intensive areas such as the intensive care unit and operating rooms.

- Equipment and Tools—Appropriate, adequate, and reliable tools are critical for the success of in-house service. Proper tools for trouble shooting and repair can cut down repair time and reduce unnecessary equipment down time. Since test equipment is used to verify the performance of medical devices, periodic calibration of test equipment in the service department should not be neglected.
- Spare Parts and Loaner Equipment—To further reduce equipment down time, an in-house service department sometimes retains one or more functional spare equipment in the department. This is often the case for high-volume or critical items. These spare equipment will be used as loaners when equipment is removed from the user's area for PM or repair. Most in-house service departments will stock frequently used spare parts, especially those that may take a long time to be shipped to the hospital.

2.1.4 Advantages and Disadvantages of In-house Service

There are many advantages of in-house service over other service modalities. Some of the obvious ones are listed below:

- There is full administrative control over the service as all staff are employed by the facility.
- Response to an equipment service call is immediate as staff is located in the facility.
- There is greater flexibility in assigning work, e.g., it is easier to change duty assignments to meet changing needs.
- There is no travel time involved, especially comparing to "parts and labor" type of service contracts where travel time is also billed to the customers.
- In-house service personnel usually have better communication and rapport with device users.
- There is always someone in the facility to answer questions and carry out minor tasks.
- In-house service is generally less expensive for the same type of work.

Although there are many advantages, in-house service does suffer from some drawbacks. Some of the disadvantages are listed below:

- The facility needs to pay for staff training.
- The facility needs to have a capital budget for test equipment and parts inventory.
- There are overhead and operating costs for the in-house service, such as clerical support, utilities, space, management, etc.
- There are limited backup resources available, including both staff and equipment.
- For small departments, skills and experience are limited.

It must be noted than when the disadvantages listed above are properly studied, many of them can be overcome. For example, the high cost of service training and software diagnostic tools can be negotiated and budgeted up front at the time of device purchase.

Perhaps the biggest concern with in-house service, especially with departments that service large capital items such as medical imaging and medical laboratory equipment, is the possibility of an unforeseeable expensive repair. While this concern is real, there are ways of managing these types of problems and minimizing the risk of large-ticket repairs. The idea of so-called "self-insurance" is a way to minimize this impact by spreading the repair cost over a large repair and maintenance budget. This concept will be discussed later.

2.2 External Service Contracts

One of the most popular methods of maintaining medical devices, especially in smaller hospitals, is through service contract agreements. These agreements between the facility and the device distributor generally come into effect after the new device warranty has expired. It is very important that facilities discuss with the vendor and agree to the terms of the service contracts (and their respective costs and additional costs) and if possible include them in the overall conditions of purchase. The facility can usually get a "better deal" as a result of the negotiation, especially when the cost of the service is rolled into one overall medical device purchasing agreement. Such considerations will also help to establish the overall operational cost of the new equipment.

One quality control indicator which may be used to determine the effectiveness of a service contract is the guarantee of equipment "uptime," that is, the percentage of time that the device will be operational and ready for use. This "uptime guarantee" and its penalty should be clearly stated in the service contract purchase agreement.

There are many different options in putting together a service contract. For instance, the hospital may contract out the work to a third-party service provider instead of purchasing service from the manufacturers. In both cases, the scope and details of the required work should be clearly stated and written into the service contract agreement before it is signed by the facility and the service provider.

2.2.1 Types of Service Contracts

Listed below are some common types of service contract arrangements, each of which may have many different variations.

1. *Full parts and labor support, also known as full service contract.* This may be the most popular, most comprehensive, yet the most expensive type of service contract. Under full service agreement, all maintenance, including preventive maintenance and repair, plus all replacement parts are included. When negotiating this type of contract, one must pay attention to the coverage hours (i.e., the hours of the day during which the service vendor will come and repair the equipment) and overtime charges. The facility must consider the department work pattern in order to determine the best option in order to reduce the service cost and to meet the operational requirements of the department.

2. *Partial parts and labor support.* This type of service contract is similar to "full service contract," and is especially popular when large capital equipment is involved such as major medical diagnostic imaging unit or medical laboratory equipment. Usually in this type of agreement, large ticket replacement items (such as X-ray tubes, ultrasound probes, etc.) and consumables are excluded from coverage, while less expensive parts and all labor are covered. It is very important to perform some analysis to determine what is the best overall package before it is signed. In order to achieve this, analysis of device usage, expected life span, frequency and cost of component replacement, typical device service requirements, etc. must be undertaken. This is where the technical expertise of an in-house clin-

ical engineer becomes invaluable, as the dollar values for servicing a sophisticated medical device such as a magnetic resonant imaging (MRI) scanner can be in the hundreds of thousands of dollars.

3. *Parts only contract.* This type of contract is typically used by facilities that have the technical expertise on the device but wish to guarantee or effectively predict the variable cost of expensive parts replacement. Parts only contracts are also popular with large-ticket items. In this case, the facility pays an annual lump sum for all the replacement parts while in-house personnel perform the service work.

4. *Labor only contract.* In contrast to parts only contract, the service vendor will perform all necessary work, but the facility will have to purchase the required replacement parts (either from the manufacturer or a second source).

5. *Time and materials.* In this contractual arrangement, service work is charged to the facility at a set labor rate, with all parts paid for by the facility as well. In a variation of this arrangement, a service provider may for a set fee provide service up to a predetermined amount of time at a lower than normal rate. The work performed above this time limit will be charged at a higher rate.

6. *Preventive maintenance contract.* In a preventive maintenance contract, the vendor provides an established number of preventive maintenance checks on the equipment per year in return for a negotiated amount of money. A permutation on this type of contract would be the inclusion of a limited number of demand maintenance, i.e., repair calls. Otherwise, repair services found in PM checks are usually charged at an established labor rate with parts paid for by the facility.

7. *Repair service, or demand maintenance contract.* This is the "opposite" to a preventive maintenance contract. In this case, repair work is covered under the contract, while in-house personnel perform the PMs. This type of contract is popular on large-capital items that cannot tolerate unscheduled lengthy downtime.

8. *Shared service contract.* Many manufacturers offer discounts on contracts in which in-house personnel perform first-line call screening and troubleshooting. Oftentimes this reduces equipment downtime by allowing in-house personnel to take care of

minor problems while still having access to full manufacturer's service support. The manufacturer can achieve savings in reducing travel by solving problems together with in-house service staff over the telephone. Quite often, in conjunction with a shared service agreement, a part consignment (i.e., selected spare parts are stored on site) is arranged to further reduce equipment down time.

2.2.2 Criteria to Consider in Negotiating Service Contracts

When negotiating a service contract, a number of factors must be taken into consideration. The facility should evaluate the service proposal as well as the service provider and take into consideration the capability and resources of the in-house service. Some requirements to look for are listed below:

- location of service personnel
- number of local service representatives
- training and experience of the local service representatives
- location of backup service
- whether service is provided by the manufacturer's employee or by a local dealer
- hourly labor rate and standard service hours
- any additional labor cost and overtime rate
- how travel time is charged
- guaranteed response time (both by telephone and on-site)
- range of replacement parts stored locally
- primary location of parts; how quickly they can be shipped
- current parts price lists (if parts are charged extra)
- credit for returning defective parts
- number of PMs provided and copies of PM procedures
- any limits on PMs and repairs
- whether or not loaner equipment is provided
- liability insurance coverage
- uptime guarantee and penalty for nonconformance

If the service is provided by a third-party service provider rather than by the device manufacturer, the facility should look at the following:

- sources of replacement parts, i.e., whether parts are from the original equipment manufacturers or substitution sources

- availability of technical information such as service manuals
- availability of diagnostic software and tools
- years in business
- references

The other consideration when negotiating contracts for facilities with an in-house BME department is the possibility of different levels of cooperative service options between the in-house service and external service provider. In any case, the facility should be cautious before signing a multiple year service agreement with a vendor as service requirements could change with time. An escape clause is recommended in the contract document.

2.2.3 Monitoring Outside Service Work

It is very important to maintain control over repair work performed on hospital equipment by external service providers, such as the manufacturer or a third-party service provider. When purchasing service contracts for equipment repair or negotiating warranty service for new equipment, one should keep in mind that, given adequate resources and technical training, in-house maintenance is usually less-expensive and more efficient.

In those few cases where external service is deemed to be a more effective solution for servicing certain pieces of equipment, it is important that these service activities are properly coordinated and managed. Without continuous monitoring of the work performed by external service providers, there is no way of ascertaining whether or not equipment is maintained at an acceptable level, i.e., serviced regularly, to specification, and to an adequate level of performance and quality. Also there is no way of ascertaining whether the performed maintenance service was necessary, sufficient, or even desirable. When using external service providers, healthcare facilities must not neglect the need to monitor and cannot assume that services provided are always of high quality and satisfactory. Qualified technical personnel should verify the work performed to ensure that the contract services are completed as outlined in the contract agreement. To achieve this, the in-house CSP should coordinate and oversee all equipment services performed by external contractors, no matter whether it is new installation, warranty work or demand maintenance.

The need to audit externally contracted work is also evident when the contracts are being renewed or new equipment is being purchased. By maintaining complete repair and service records for medical equipment, subsequent renewal of service contracts can be more closely scrutinized to ensure that the facility is achieving the most cost-effective use of its maintenance dollar. Also, the documented service history of a service provider may contain useful information that is useful at equipment purchase time, or may indicate which manufacturers or vendors to avoid.

External contract works must also be fully documented similar to in-house performed services. A special database to keep track of device service contracts and service history is essential. The database should record what service contracts are purchased, what equipment falls under the jurisdiction of the service contracts, as well as other information regarding the details of the contracts. Statistics related to the service histories of devices covered is helpful to evaluate the cost-effectiveness of the contract. To capture this information, details of the service rendered, such as repairs time, travel time, parts costs, problem descriptions, and corrective actions must all be recorded in the database. Such an equipment management record keeping system will be discussed later in another chapter.

2.2.4 Advantages and Disadvantages of External Service Contracts

Some of the advantages of service contracts over other service modalities are listed below:
- There is no need to arrange specialized (sometimes expensive) technical training to in-house staff.
- The costs of equipment maintenance are known for budgetary purpose.
- The possibility of incurring a large repair expense is eliminated.
- A qualified vendor should be able to fix any device problem and is obligated under contract to do so at no additional cost to the facility.
- Downtime is usually lower as replacement parts are most likely in stock at the manufacturer's service depot.
- The work performed by the device manufacturer is usually of high quality.

Despite the above advantages, there are many disadvantages of external service contracts. Many have been discussed in previous sections in this chapter, below are a few obvious ones:

- There are numerous extra built-in costs with service contracts, making them inherently more expensive than in-house service. For example, the travel time involved for the service personnel to come to the facility is always billed to the customer either at a travel rate or built into the cost of a lump sum contract.
- Response to a service call is not immediate due to travelling. Excessive lengthy equipment down time is possible when there are too many simultaneous service calls from different customers

Even though the external service providers performing the maintenance work are technically competent, there still exists the need to have someone involved in monitoring the service activities in the facility. Proper management of service contracts is critical to a technology management program. Too many facilities, however, find themselves without proper control over their maintenance expenses due to the lack of in-house technical knowledge. Technical auditing to ensure compliance with minimum standards is a must to ensure that the facility is getting the service it pays for.

2.3 Maintenance Insurance and Self-insurance

Maintenance insurance by its name is a form of insurance. Instead of paying for someone to perform the service, a healthcare facility may choose to pay a fixed premium to an insurance company. In return, the insurance company will pay for all the associated costs to maintain the insured equipment during the insured period. In most cases, when there is a need to service a device, the healthcare facility will initiate the service call either to the insurance company or to an authorized service provider. In the former case, the insurance company will then call the appropriate service provider. The service provider who performed the work may be paid directly by the insurance company, or paid by the healthcare facility that will later be reimbursed by the insurance company. It should be noted that a full-service contract is in effect a form of maintenance insurance; in this case, the service provider who offers the service contract is the insurer. Some advantages to the healthcare facility of using maintenance insurance are:

- Fix expenditure in terms of device maintenance. Ideal for budgeting.
- Healthcare facilities do not need to worry about unexpected

high repair cost.
- It may be cheaper (as claimed by maintenance insurance providers) than purchasing service contracts.

When considering a maintenance insurance proposal, the healthcare facility should consider the following potential problems:
- The healthcare facility may not have a choice of who will provide the service. The insurance company usually selects the service provider.
- There may be undesirable lengthy downtime if the third party service provider does not have the expertise or replacement parts to render the service.
- Maintenance insurance providers often require users to keep extensive documentation.
- It may create labor-intensive and complicated documentation and invoicing processes.
- Free software upgrade, which is often provided as part of the service contract, will not be available.
- Insurance premium will rise in subsequent years if the service expenditure is excessive.

Instead of paying a maintenance insurance premium to a private insurance provider, some hospitals have grouped together to provide "self-insurance" to their group members. The principle of self-insurance is based on the fact that a large maintenance pool formed by multiple hospitals can more readily absorb an unpredicted expensive repair bill than the maintenance budget of a single hospital. In one example, four hospitals located in close geographical area joined together to form a self-insurance program. Each member hospital pays a predetermined annual premium to a central maintenance pool. Any expenses related to device maintenance are drawn from the pool. The formula to determine the annual contribution and hence the premium is reviewed periodically.

2.4 Contracted Technology Management

Even though a healthcare facility has purchased maintenance insurance for all its medical technology, there is still a need for an in-house person (or a group of individuals) to coordinate the service activities. Another option of maintenance modality is contracted technology (or equipment) management. Under such arrangement, the provider will have a manager and service personnel stationed in the facility to provide the necessary equipment management functions including equipment service. From the user's perspective, contracted technology management may have little difference from normal in-house service other than the fact that the service providers are no longer employees of the facility. Depending on the agreement (and of course, the cost), contracted equipment management may provide total technology management function to the facility.

It is important to understand that private companies that offer service contracts, maintenance insurance, or contracted technology management programs are all trying to profit from the agreements. In theory, a properly run in-house service department will always achieve better savings and provide a better quality of service.

3 REGIONAL SUPPORT MODELS

3.1 Shared Service Agreements

To establish an in-house Biomedical Engineering Department requires considerable investment in terms of facilities and human resources. For small-sized hospitals, it may not be cost-effective to have their own in-house service department. It should be obvious that it is difficult to find a technologist who has the expertise in all areas of medical technology (radiology, monitoring equipment, and laboratory instrumentation, etc). Regional shared service is an option to provide comprehensive services to smaller healthcare facilities. Larger centers can also benefit from a shared service arrangement in terms of economy of scale and resources sharing. Below are three possible organizations of regional services:

1. Jointly owned and administered by two or more facilities. For example, several hospitals jointly fund a Biomedical Engineering Department. The department manager reports to a committee composed of representatives from each of the hospitals.

2. Purchase service by one facility from another. For example, a small hospital purchases the service from a nearby larger medical center.

3. Sharing resources. For example, two nearby hospitals, A and B, both have their own in-house BME department. An agreement

is signed to provide backup services and to share expensive, infrequently used test equipment. In addition, hospital A supports the diagnostic imaging equipment in hospital B and hospital B supports the medical laboratory equipment in hospital A.

Based on the circumstances, a combination of the above can be arranged to better fit the characteristics and the needs of the facilities.

3.2 Advantages and Disadvantages of Regional Shared Support

The advantages of a regional shared service arrangement are listed below:

- Shared service is usually less expensive than an external service contract.
- Better negotiating power in service contract procurement due to the economy of scale.
- Able to share expensive test equipment.
- Can reduce overall training cost.
- Will maintain a more stable organization due to a bigger pool of staff.
- May increase efficiency from specialization.
- May decrease overhead.

However, in considering a shared service arrangement, a facility should be aware of the following pitfalls:

- Increase in non-productive time (e.g., time spent in travelling).
- Potential dispute in the shared cost and services received.
- Sense of commitment of individual staff members may be compromised.
- More difficult for managers to supervise staff members.
- Expertise may not be available when needed (when a particular individual is at another facility).

To maintain a regional shared service arrangement, unless it is a purchased service, it is important that:

- Appropriate resources are allocated to the service.
- All users are in favor of the arrangement.
- There is a fair and agreed cost sharing formula.
- There is a steering committee with representation from all participating facilities to oversee the operation of the service.
- There are mechanisms to periodically review and improve the performance and structure of the service.

Chapter 5

TECHNOLOGY ACCEPTANCE
AND DOCUMENTATION

1 INCOMING INSPECTION AND COMMISSIONING

An important first step in technology management is to ensure that all technology brought into a healthcare environment is safe and effective. In order to achieve this goal, it is necessary to ensure that every piece of medical equipment has passed an incoming safety and performance inspection before it is used in patient care areas. All medical equipment, whether on loan, on evaluation, donated, leased, or bought by the hospital or by individual health care providers, must be inspected. The purpose of the inspection is fourfold:

- to ensure than the device meets its minimum performance

requirements, as specified in the performance specifications.
- to verify that all components and accessories listed in the purchase order (PO) are received in good order.
- to ensure that the device meets all regulatory requirements including safety standards.
- to establish a reference level of device performance. Such reference is used to compare against subsequent performance verification results.

1.1 Incoming Inspection

The usual tests performed on the equipment during incoming inspection may be divided into the following categories:
1. visual inspections
2. verification of appropriate labeling (e.g., CE marking) and regulatory approval (e.g., CSA approval)
3. safety inspection, e.g., electrical safety tests on electrical-powered devices
4. verification of performance
5. account for all items (including documentation) specified in the PO

Qualified in-house individuals, such as members of the Biomedical Engineering Department, are to perform these inspections. To ensure that all items purchased are inspected and crossed referenced to the purchasing requirements, a complete purchase order must accompany the equipment to be inspected. The results of these tests must be recorded in an incoming inspection form and placed in the device record file. After the incoming inspection is completed and the device is accepted for use in the facility, the device should be added to the medical equipment inventory database.

The incoming inspection process is shown in Figure 5–1. The vendor will be notified to rectify the deficiencies for any failure in the inspection process. Devices which passed the inspections will be added to the inventory and deployed to the clinical areas.

1.2 Commissioning

Commissioning refers to the initial testing and performance verification of an installation or system when it is first installed. Commis-

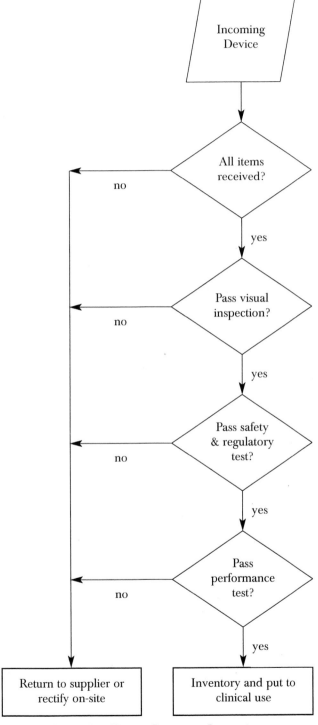

Figure 5–1. Device Incoming Inspection.

sioning is in fact incoming inspection of a large or complicated system. Its purpose is to make sure that the device or system performs according to the design specifications and operates satisfactory in the clinical environment. For a complex system or large capital installation, it may be beyond the capability of an individual or a single in-house department to perform the inspection. In that case, a team from several disciplines is needed to perform the task. A third-party expert may be employed to commission a large installation on behalf of the hospital, such as a new medical gas supply system. In addition to providing technical expertise, third-party commissioning will also provide an independent assessment of the system before making the final acceptance by the hospital.

2 INVENTORY MANAGEMENT AND DOCUMENTATION

Probably the single most important element to ensure successful management of medical devices in a healthcare facility is an accurate, up-to-date and comprehensive inventory of all medical equipment in the facility. Upon completion of the incoming inspection, a device record file should be created and should remain active throughout the useful life span of the equipment. The device is identified and tracked by an equipment control number (ECN). The ECN is a unique number assigned and tagged onto the medical device right after it has passed the incoming inspection. In addition to the ECN, the device record file records such information as the equipment purchase information, ownership and user information, warranty and service history, etc.

The device record file should also contain the service history of the equipment, including the results of every preventive maintenance inspection, repair services, and if available, device modifications. It documents work performed by in-house maintenance staff as well as warranty and demand maintenance done by suppliers and outside service contractors. Nowadays, most in-house BME Departments are keeping this information in a computerized equipment management system, although some still keep paper records for security and liability reasons.

To ensure that a medical device is suitable for use in a particular procedure and clinical environment, it needs to be appropriately labeled. A service label with the date of last service and date of next service should be attached visibly on the medical equipment. Equipment that is not suitable for use in an area or not fit to be used should be removed and properly labeled to ensure that it will not be inadvertently put back into service. Furthermore, the status and service record of the device should be kept up-to-date in the device record file and database.

2.1 Requirements of a Medical Equipment Management Database

A medical equipment management database is a vital tool for managing technology effectively and efficiently. It also serves as a source of information for the daily maintenance activities. The main functions of such a system are:
- maintain equipment inventory
- record service history
- track service requests
- schedule preventive maintenance
- maintain and track replacement parts inventory
- generate equipment management reports

Below is a list of the basic elements that the database system should contain:
- an equipment control number (ECN)
- a generic description of the equipment, preferably conforming to the industry-accepted ECRI nomenclature
- the equipment manufacturer, model number, and serial number
- the owner department and/or cost center number
- the normal location of the equipment
- the purchase order number and date
- the equipment's acquisition cost
- the supplier's name, address, and telephone number
- the warranty conditions and expiration date
- an abbreviated description of the inspection and preventive maintenance (PM) requirements and intervals
- information regarding any applicable service contracts, e.g., vendor name, address, and telephone number, purchase order number, cost, terms, expiration date
- the location of the equipment's user and service manuals

- an abbreviated service history
- the service technologist assigned to service to device
- other pertinent information regarding the equipment, e.g., sources of critical parts

An example of a medical device record form is shown in Figure 5–2. The technologist responsible for the device incoming inspection is responsible to complete the form and enter the information into the medical equipment management system to start tracking the device.

The database is important to the day-to-day operations and management activities of the technology management program. As such, it is important that the database demonstrates as a minimum the following four characteristics:

1. The database must be complete, accurate and current. The responsibility to up keep the information lies with the centralized service provider (e.g., the BME Department).

2. The database must be readily available and easy to use so that the service provider is able to immediately ascertain the status of the device, access parts inventories, and recall the device's service history.

3. The database must be well documented and flexible to allow

---

BIOMEDICAL ENGINEERING
MEDICAL DEVICE RECORD

ID NUMBER (ECN) _____   DESCRIPTION _____

MANUFACTURER _____   MODEL NUMBER _____

DEPARTMENT _____ COST CENTRE _____   SERIAL NUMBER _____

LOCATION _____   STATUS _____

PURCHASE VENDOR _____   SERVICE CONTRACT NUMBER _____

PURCHASE COST _____ DATE _____   CONTRACT EXPIRY DATE _____

PO NUMBER _____   PARTS VENDOR _____

WARRANTY EXPIRY DATE _____   SERVICE MANUAL NUMBER _____

PM PRIORITY _____ PM PROCEDURE _____   TECHNOLOGIST _____

Figure 5–2. Medical Device Record.

the department manager to generate reports on a wide range of technology management activities, including generating statistics and quality indicators.

4. The system should be versatile and easily modifiable in order to handle changing demands.

It is also desirable that the database be an integral part or linked to the hospital's computerized information system (HIS) so that medical equipment information (e.g., status, service records, etc.) can be viewed, shared, or retrieved by others (e.g., equipment users, accounting personnel, etc.). Although some hospitals may choose to develop their own computer program, database software specifically designed for this purpose is available. Examples of some off-the-shelf programs are: the "Profile" by Biotek (http://www.biotekbiomedical.com) and the "Hospital Equipment Control System (HECS)" by ECRI (http://www.ecri.org). Most of these computer programs include a replacement parts inventorying system, which can be used with the equipment database to automatically determine service costs, parts availability, parts ordering information, etc.

In addition to documenting service activities, most computerized medical equipment management systems can generate PM service schedules and some can prioritize maintenance activities based on equipment profiles and service histories.

2.2 Management Information

Not only is the medical equipment management database useful in efficiently supporting service activities such as work scheduling and parts ordering, much useful management information can be made available from the database system. Such information is crucial to supporting various aspects of technology management, some of which include:

- equipment replacement planning
- facility-wide equipment standardization
- determining cross-charges and technology costs for individual departments
- tracking maintenance costs for devices or user areas in order to ascertain exceptionally high cost areas
- computation of service request response time
- manpower planning, specifically of biomedical engineering

technologist resource requirements, a shortage of which could manifest itself as excessive equipment downtime

- tracking problems with specific devices, which could indicate equipment abuse or lack of user training, e.g., too many "operator errors"
- tracking equipment work histories for use on device replacement decisions
- risk management activities, such as hazard alert tracking, actions planning, and monitoring

2.3 Supplies and Parts Inventory Management

Most medical devices require accessories and consumable parts. For example, an ECG monitor needs disposable electrodes to acquire the patient's electrocardiogram; the x-ray tube of a CT scanner needs to be replaced after about 60,000 scans; the patient breathing circuit of an anesthesia machine needs to be replaced after every patient use.

Based on usage, there are three major categories of supplies and parts for medical devices. They are operational accessories and supplies, service consumable parts and supplies, and demand maintenance replacement parts.

2.3.1 Operational Accessories and Supplies

These are attachments and parts that are needed for the normal operation of the medical device. ECG cables and leads, infusion sets, and patient breathing circuits are some examples. Supplies can be single use, i.e., disposable, or multiple use, i.e., reusable. Manufacturers of the medical supplies always specify whether their products are single or multiple use. The labeling of such information is required by regulatory agencies (such as FDA) to be imprinted on the package of the product.

2.3.2 Service Consumables

Service consumable parts and supplies are components or items, often inside the device, that are subject to wear and tear or depletion under normal use. Examples are calibration gas in an anesthetic gas monitor and the x-ray tube in a CT scanner. Some of the medical devices are designed to provide indications to the users when the consumables need to be replaced or replenished. Other will rely on the users' experience to initiate the replacement. For some devices, the users are required to perform routine inspections and periodically replace or replenish the consumable items. A thorough PM procedure always includes checking service consumable items.

2.3.3 Demand Maintenance Replacement Parts

These are components to replace faulty items during troubleshooting and repairs. Experienced service personnel are able to identify common failure items and appropriately keep them in stock to facilitate repair and therefore reduce equipment down time.

The BME Department usually is responsible for service consumables and repair replacement parts. Medical accessories and supplies are ordered by the Purchasing Department and stocked by the Central Stores. Processing (cleaning, disinfection, sterilization, etc.) of reusable items is done by the Central Supplies Department.

Due to economic reasons, some hospitals are reusing "single use supplies." Studies have shown that some supplies that are labeled as "single use" can be used multiple times without either losing their effectiveness or imposing additional risk to patients provided that they are processed properly after every use. Reusing dialyzers in hemodialysis is a good example. When making a decision to reuse a "single use item," it is important to perform a hazard analysis and evaluate the associated savings. Some hospitals have a "Reuse Committee" to review and approve every reuse request. Many of these committees are also responsible to establish policies and procedures governing reuse of "single use supplies." More information about reuse can be found in the Proceedings of the Symposium on "Reuse of Disposable Medical Devices" held in 1994 in Montreal, Canada (http://www.ccohta.ca).

As there are many, and often too many, medical supplies in a health care facility, they require tremendous resources to acquire, store, process, deliver, and track. It makes sense to reduce the number of different devices in the facility in order to reduce the number of medical supplies. The primary role of the "Product Standardization Committee" is to reduce the number of different brands and models of medical devices and therefore minimize their supplies in the facility. For example, only one model of general infusion pump is used throughout the facility. Therefore, only a few types of infusion sets are stocked in the hospital. Some advantages of standardizing product are listed below:

- Reduce user-training requirements
- Simplify parts inventory
- Improve utilization by pooling a smaller number of devices
- Able to negotiate volume discount on supplies
- Reduce service down time by borrowing from low use area

2.4 Service Documentation

The information gathered from medical device management activities such as PM or corrective maintenance (CM) is essential for many of the performance and quality audit functions of a medical technology management program. In order to support this, the following policies must be in place:

1. An inventory of all medical equipment, including a comprehensive and complete work history, is to be established and maintained.
2. All medical equipment in the healthcare facility is to be placed on an inspection schedule.
3. Procedures for performing preventive maintenance for all medical equipment in the facility are to be developed and implemented.
4. Mechanisms for reporting equipment services are to be established.

An equipment service work order should be created and remained open once a service requisition is received. In order to track the cost of equipment maintenance and to ensure that information is available to substantiate capital equipment replacement planning, all service work performed on equipment must be reported. Documentation formats for PM, CM, and service requisitions were discussed in Chapter 3.

The service history of individual equipment or a group of equipment of the same makes and models can reveal useful technical information such as failure rates and trends. For examples, repeated service requests with no problem found could indicate an intermittent problem; too many operator errors indicate a need for user training. Many requests for service and, more significantly, many equipment-related injuries are usually the results of user errors as opposed to equipment malfunction. The Joint Commission on Accreditation of Healthcare Organizations (JCAHO) *Accreditation Manual for Hospitals* requires that all operator errors be identified, documented, and reviewed by the safety committee. In this way, trends can be identified on a particular device or class of devices to avoid potential problems.

Independent of whether the BME department works on a charge-back system or not, the cost of the service should be recorded on the service report. The inventory report may then keep a running tab on the cost of the equipment's maintenance and provide valuable information for other quality audit determinations.

In addition to allowing individual departments to meet accreditation rules, it is necessary to develop and formalize a mechanism whereby summaries of equipment service activities in each of the service areas are periodically reported back to the department. The frequencies and contents of the summary report are usually established between the area and the centralized service provider (e.g., between the Operating Room and BMED). Common reporting items include number of repairs, number of PM, total labor to perform the services, cost of replacement parts, etc. Such statistics can also be used for quality assurance purposes of the technology management system.

Chapter 6

RISK MANAGEMENT, EDUCATION
AND QUALITY ASSURANCE

1 RISK MANAGEMENT

1.1 Essential Components of a Risk Management Program

Hazard is a condition that could jeopardize safety and is therefore a source of potential danger. Risk measures the probability and severity of loss or injury. Risk management is a proactive approach to identify and correct problems. It includes prediction of injury, avoidance of exposure to hazards, and minimization of liability. This section introduces how we can reduce risks associated with medical technology through implementation of a risk management program.

The Canadian Council of Health Facility Accreditation (CCHFA), in its accreditation standards, defined risk management as "a systematic process of identifying, assessing and taking action to prevent or manage clinical, administrative, property and occupational health and safety risks in the facility." Compromising the designed performance of a medical technology through abuse or neglect can have a significant negative impact on the safety and quality of patient care. Manufacturers, when designing medical equipment, can rarely foresee each and every potential hazardous condition that may arise when the device is used in the clinical environment. Risk management is therefore an integral part of a technology management program in any healthcare facility to ensure a safe environment.

Among all the activities in a medical technology risk management program, the following are considered crucial towards a hazard-free environment:

1. hazard report management
2. incident investigation
3. user in-service education
4. medical device performance assurance inspection
5. device and product prepurchase evaluation

Preventive maintenance and performance assurance inspection was covered in Chapter 3. Device and product prepurchase evaluation will be discussed in detail later in the book. This section will concentrate primarily on items 1, 2, and 3.

1.2 Hazard Report Management

Healthcare facilities receive, through a variety of "doorways," notifications of defective or hazardous medical products including medical devices and their accessories. Some information sources report device-related problems as well as user precautions. These sources include regulatory bodies, trade journals, product manufacturers, in-house users, service personnel, and other nonprofit organizations such as the Emergency Care Research Institute (ECRI) in the United States.

For a serious problem, medical devices may be recalled. A recall may involve removal of the device from service permanently or temporarily for modification or repair. Once a problem has been identified (e.g., design defect or inaccurate labeling), the manufacturer is obligated to notify all the users. Under such circumstances, the manufacturer may be responsible for repairing the defective device, replacing it, or refunding all or part of the purchase cost. If a hospital continued to use a device after receiving a recall or hazard notification and subsequently caused an injury, the hospital may be held liable. Therefore it is important that an effective mechanism is in place to manage all these notifications.

In order to properly manage hazard reports, the following must be established within the facility.

1.2.1 Policies and Procedures

In any hospitals, device users may respond to hazard alerts in different ways. They may distribute the reports to other users or circulate them only within their areas. There must exist facility-wide policies and procedures to direct staff on how to receive, distribute, follow-up, and document hazard reports and recall notices.

1.2.2 Coordination of Activities

Any department or individual within the facility may receive hazard reports directly from outside sources. To properly manage hazard reporting, a centralized body must be assigned the responsibility of coordinating the functions. Without proper coordination, some reports may never be delivered to the affected areas, and hence hazardous situations may never be acted upon or be rectified. It is desirable to assign one person within a facility to coordinate such activities. The coordinator must have the following attributes:
- have a general knowledge of hospital products and equipment
- be familiar with the hospital system and the functions of different healthcare teams within the hospital
- understand the nature of risks associated with products and equipment
- be a member of the quality or risk management committees within the facility

• have a clearly defined role and authority within the risk management program

The Purchasing Department, which handles the acquisition and initial distribution of all hospital equipment and supplies, is one of the logical bodies to coordinate the hazard report management activities. The Biomedical Engineering Department, which is the technical expert in medical device technology, is another group that can assume this lead role. In any case, the Hazard Report Management Coordinator must work with both Purchasing and Biomedical Engineering to ensure that all reports are thoroughly reviewed, appropriately distributed, and promptly acted upon.

1.2.3 Documentation

One important aspect of a risk management program is to ensure that all information received and all actions taken are fully documented until the hazardous problem is resolved. Thorough documentation is critical to ensure the completion of all appropriate responses. A well-documented hazard report management program is the best defense in potential liability litigation. In addition, useful technology management information can be derived from the hazard documentation (e.g., information to assist in equipment replacement planning).

1.2.4 Tracking Mechanism

Once a notification of hazard has been received by the hospital, a follow-up mechanism must be in place to initiate corrective actions and to ensure that affected users have been notified. Since many of the problems may be beyond the capability of one individual to handle, there is a potential danger that inappropriate decisions could be made. For example, a user might not be aware of the seriousness of an intermittent problem and not consult other hospital professionals. The coordinator plays a critical role in centralizing all incoming hazard notifications and distributing them to the affected areas.

A hazard report management program with a proper follow-up mechanism and a comprehensive documentation requirement will reveal trends and common problems to help reducing risks. Table 6–1 shows the summary table of a hazard report management program to help to track the progress of hazard notifications that have been determined to affect devices in the hospital. The detailed documentation of hazard notifications and their follow-up actions are stored in files identified by the hazard report identification number (HRID).

Table 6–1

SUMMARY OF HAZARD REPORT MANAGEMENT

HRID Date	Source Ref.	Summary of hazard	Parties Notified	Actions	Follow-up	Status
HD0892 01/15/01	OR Staff	Gas leakage from O2 E-cylinder yoke	OR, RT	BMED investigating		Active
HD0893 12/20/00	ECRI 32-243	HP M2000 HR alarm failure	CCU, ICU, EMERG	Warning labels applied on units. Vendor notified 10/01/00	01/03/01	Active
HD0894 09/07/00	Health Canada MDA-113	Cleaning of reusable resuscitators and PEEP valves	RT, CSD	See MDA-113-A1 in file	10/21/00 11/04/00	Closed

1.3 Incident Investigation

ECRI, in their Hospital Risk Control Information and Consulting System, defines an incident as "any occurrence out of the ordinary which may involve risk or actual injury to an individual or damage to hospital property." Examples of common incidents in hospitals are patient falls and medication errors. As medical devices become more integrated into the provision of health care, the frequency of medical device-related incidents has inevitably increased. Medical device-related incidents include:

1. any apparent malfunction, misuse, or failure of medical devices, supplies, and hospital facilities which adversely affected the quality of care or the safety of patients or staff;
2. any events in which a patient is suddenly injured or dies unexpectedly while connected to a medical device;

3. any events which have involved medical devices and have resulted in the generation of a hospital incident report.

Many health care facilities have developed policies and established mechanisms for reporting and investigating incidents. The primary purpose is to identify the cause of the problem and take appropriate action in order to minimize the possibility of a similar future incident. Other purposes of incident investigation and reporting are:

- To provide administrators, managers, clinical staff, and other relevant personnel with prompt and factual information about incidents.
- In the event of litigation, to provide an accessible and accurate documentation of the incident, subsequent investigation, and remedial action.
- Investigation of medical-device related incidents may provide manufacturers with constructive feedback in design problems.
- To report medical device problems to regulatory agencies.

An incident should be investigated immediately after its occurrence. An investigation team should be setup to formally investigate a serious incident. The team should be composed of managers of the user departments, the hospital's Quality and Risk Coordinator, and other people who can contribute to the investigation. For all medical device-related incidents, the Biomedical Engineering Department must be involved. The investigation should be thoroughly documented and should focus on fact-finding rather than to identify whom is to blame.

While conducting an investigation of an incident involving medical devices, the following priorities should be kept in mind:

- Remove the possibility of further injury to the patients.
- Attend to the immediate needs of the patients.
- Prevent further damages to medical devices and the facilities.
- Impound devices that may be hazardous or are suspected to have caused the incident.
- Determine the sequence of events that took place during the incident.

During the investigation, the following procedures should be followed:

- The person taking the initial call from the clinical area should record the name of the caller, time of the incident, type of incident, and the patient condition.

- The clinical area should be advised not to disturb the equipment and accessories if possible.
- An incident investigation team should be formed.
- The team should interview clinical staff who witnessed the incident, take notes during the interview, and consciously separate the facts from the opinion.
- All medical devices and accessories implicated in the incident should be inspected and the results documented.
- From the information gathered, determine the possible cause of the incident and suggest remedial actions.
- Consult with the affected clinical areas regarding impacts due to the remedial action.
- Once the cause of the incident is determined, the remedial action should be implemented as quickly as possible.
- Notify the clinical staff when the remedial action is complete.
- Complete and file the incident investigation report.

In order to achieve the goal of investigating incidents properly and taking appropriate actions, perhaps the most critical issue to be considered is that of staff awareness. Once again, all hospital staff must be aware of the incident reporting policies and practices in the hospital. Even with awareness of the policies and procedures, hospital staff must be trained and reminded on how to recognize and report incidents. The question of determining what constitutes an incident is also an issue that must be addressed at staff training sessions.

The development of a policy and procedure regarding incident investigation should include the development of an incident investigation form to capture all relevant information during the investigation. A copy of the report is appended to the end of this chapter. The policy and procedure should include a mechanism to circulate and review incident investigation reports.

1.4 Technology Education

While technology education may sound remote from medical device risk management, it is one of the first steps toward accident prevention. Data gathered from 1986 to 1989 through the "Device Adverse Experience Network," published by the U.S. Bureau of Radiation and Medical Devices, indicates that user misunderstanding and techniques was the cause for about 16 percent of the reported problems. ECRI reported that about 40 percent of all medical device service requests are related to improper use.

The Canadian Council of Health Facilities Accreditation (CCHFA) standards, and similar bodies in other countries, requires hospitals to have a staff development program in place. These programs are man-dated towards attaining and maintaining staff's competencies in their areas of practice. The Canadian Standards Association (CSA) standard on "Electrical Safety in Patient Care Areas," CAN/CSA-Z32.2-M89, section 4.4.1, stated that "Education programs shall be delivered to operators and technical staff. These programs shall include (a) hazards awareness of equipment both to the operators and the patients; (b) contraindications for use of specific equipment with a specific patient; and (c) basic operational maintenance requirements of equipment." Furthermore, "the Special Report on Medical Device and the Law," published by ECRI (*Health Technology,* Vol. 3 No. 3, Fall 1989), alleged that "failure to operate equipment in accordance with instructions may shift liability from the manufacturer to the user . . . most equipment-related incidents result from equipment misuse or user error . . . edu-cating users is paramount to avoiding equipment-related incidents."

In order to successfully manage risk and to provide a hazard free environment, both initial and ongoing user in-service education are essential. The best people to define user-training requirements are the users themselves. The same set of requirements should apply to simi-lar equipment types and be consistent across clinical units. There should be a facility-wide policy and guidelines stipulating criteria and training requirements on staff's professional development. No matter viewing from the legal, quality improvement, or risk management per-spective, there is a definite need for a unified approach to document these in-service training activities. The documentation format should be designed to facilitate continuous monitoring and assessment. More importantly, the hospital should recognize such effort by providing appropriate resources to support these activities.

To identify the needs of training (and technology support require-ments), the facility must establish guidelines to ensure that training issues are considered in the capital equipment planning and acquisi-tion process. As biomedical engineers or technologists are familiar with the theory of operation and potential hazards of medical devices, they need to be actively involved in providing device in-service train-ing to technology users. Given sufficient resources, BMED can be a resource to the clinical instructors on in-service training and technology education activities. In-service training can be divided into two main categories.

1.4.1 In-service Training of New Technology

Once a new piece of medical equipment has passed the incoming inspection, the users must become familiar and develop confidence in operating the equipment. A qualified person designated by the manufacturer should conduct the in-service training of a new technology. Training should be available to all personnel involved in the use of the new technology and should cover all components of the system. Refresher training sessions should also be provided to existing staff periodically. These refresher sessions can be provided by clinical instructors or trained individuals within the hospital.

1.4.2 General Technology Training

All clinical staff should be familiar with the hazards of electricity in the clinical environment. They should know how to protect themselves and their patients from electrical shock and be familiar with general safety procedures for handling all electro-medical equipment. In the same line, clinical staff should understand fire safety and safety precautions when handling hazardous materials. A mandatory basic introduction to these topics is to be included in the orientation sessions of new staff. Furthermore, refresher courses should be made available to all staff members. Staff members who participate in hazardous procedures must receive specific training on the technology. An example is laser safety training for nurses who handle laser equipment during laser surgical procedures.

For the purpose of quality assurance and risk management, all of these training sessions must be documented. The documentation should include who conducted the training, who attended, and when the training took place. This will provide a means of monitoring the effectiveness of the training. Another important reason to document training activities is to satisfy the risk management requirements in the technology management program. Such documentation is often required by regulatory and accreditation bodies.

Similar to the equipment control database used to track medical equipment in the system, a database or recording system is required to track all types of incidents, injuries, and adverse outcomes of care for each individual piece of equipment. Such database may provide the technology management personnel and administration with the following benefits:

- make documentation available for investigation in case of litigation
- help meet requirements that all records be kept and made available to accreditation surveyors
- ease of implementing internal audits to identify potential risks
- ease of developing and providing training and education programs for staff to reduce hazards and potential for losses to the hospital
- ease of reviewing incident reports from an equipment user's perspective
- provide valuable evidence of the needs for corrective and/or preventive actions, as well as a basis for establishing maintenance priorities
- reduce insurance cost due to better management of risk

1.5 Medical Device Problem Reporting

As discussed earlier, medical device distributors and manufacturers as well as regulatory agencies can initiate medical device alerts and recalls. In many countries, device suppliers and users are required to document all problems and report to regulatory agencies regarding any device-related incidents (e.g., under "Mandatory Problem Reporting" in the Canadian Medical Devices Regulations). Upon receiving a notification, the regulatory agency will review the nature of the incident to determine appropriate actions. Such requirements are in place to ensure that devices sold and used in the country are safe and effective. In a design problem recall, the manufacturer may perform field modifications or retrieve the product to rectify the problem.

2 QUALITY IMPROVEMENT

2.1 Definition of Quality

"Quality" refers to the ability of a product or service to meet or exceed the written or agreed upon expectation of the customers. It is a measure of satisfaction of the customers with the product or service. Examples of such expectation are price, service response, etc.

2.2 Quality Improvement

Quality programs are established to ensure that an organization achieves quality in the most effective and efficient way. A fundamental requirement for the establishment of any quality program is the ability to measure the quality of products or services provided. Without this ability, it will be impossible for the managers to understand, to monitor, and to improve quality.

The two foundations of quality improvement are customer satisfaction and management by facts. A quality improvement program should establish an attitude to put the needs of the customer in the first place. In addition, it should empower all employees to manage work that they do by collecting objective data and making informative decisions. Figure 6–1 shows the framework of a quality improvement program. A quality improvement program must include the processes of planning, implementation, monitoring, and evaluation.

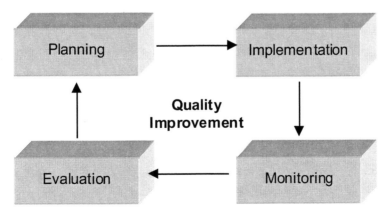

Figure 6–1. Framework of a Quality Improvement Program.

2.3 Continuous Quality Improvement

Quality improvement in a health care facility is an ongoing institutional-wide process. It provides an environment which fosters continuous risk reduction and improvement of patient care. A well-designed and implemented continuous quality improvement (CQI) program will involve staff at all levels and empower them to make changes that improve service outcomes. CQI is a philosophy and methodology focusing on continuous assessment of performance and improvement of processes. It emphasizes "structure" (i.e., defining goals and establishing policies and procedures), "process" (i.e., understanding of the operation and able to identify opportunities for improvement), and is "outcome-based" (i.e., evaluating the outcomes based on the results of pre-selected performance indicators). Figure 6–2 shows the emphasis of a CQI program.

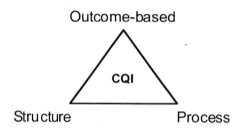

Figure 6–2. CQI Emphasis.

The enabling tasks of a CQI program are listed below:
- Assign responsibility
- Delineate scope of service
- Identify important aspects of service
- Identify key indicators
- Establish criteria for evaluation
- Collect and organize data
- Evaluate service
- Take action to solve problems
- Assess actions and document improvement
- Communicate relevant information

A CQI program for medical technology should encompasses all phases of the technology life cycle. It is a continuous structured approach designed with the goals to increase cost-effective technology utilization, ensure optimal device function, and eliminate device-related incidents.

2.4 Key Performance Indicators

A critical task in building an effective CQI Program is to establish a set of key performance indicators (KPI) to evaluate the outcomes (product or service) of the program. The first step to establish KPI is to review the goals and objectives of the program. From the goals and objectives, the CQI team identifies the program functions, the customers and their expectations. From each of these expectations, several KPI are then generated (Fig. 6–3). These indicators, once established, are used as yardsticks for quality monitoring and evaluation. To facilitate evaluation, performance thresholds or criteria are often predetermined for these indicators. A criterion violation will trigger an action to restore or improve quality. The periodic review and fine-tuning of the goals, objectives, functions, customers, expectations, and KPI are an important part of a CQI Program.

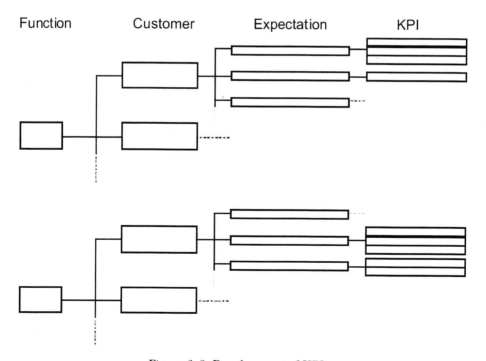

Figure 6–3. Development of KPI.

Figure 6–4 shows an example of the goals, objectives, and KPI established for a medical device incoming inspection program.

Medical Device Incoming Inspection Program

Goals

• Ensure safety of all patients and medical staff when using medical devices in any clinical area at any time.

Objectives

• Ensure that all incoming medical devices are evaluated according to established safety policies and procedures.
• Ensure that all devices entering the hospital are recorded in the medical technology management database so that they are being properly maintained.

Functions

1. Equipment evaluation
2. Incoming inspection
3. Device inventory

Customers

• Clinical device users
• Hospital buyers (Purchasing Department)
• Hospital QA Coordinator

Customer Expectations

• Evaluation to ensure that device meets clinical requirements and regulatory approval
• Inspection to ensure all items are received in good working conditions
• Fast turnaround time for incoming inspection
• Devices are accurately inventoried

Key Performance Indicators

• The number of completed device evaluations
• The number of outstanding device evaluations that are older than one month
• The number of incoming inspections performed by the in-house service department
• The percentage of new or replacement equipment coming into the hospital which requires modifications or repairs in order to pass the criteria
• The percentage of new or replacement equipment coming into the hospital which does not possess the required regulatory approval
• The number of devices that were not recorded in the medical technology management database
• The number of device records that contain missing information

---

Figure 6–4. KPI Example.

Figure 6–5

MEDICAL DEVICE INCIDENT INVESTIGATION FORM

**BIOMEDICAL ENGINEERING DEPARTMENT
CONFIDENTIAL FOR QA PURPOSES ONLY**

MEDICAL DEVICE INCIDENT INVESTIGATION FORM

INCIDENT REPORT INFORMATION	Incident Location	Incident Date (D/M/Y) / /	Incident Time (0000) HOURS	Patient Injuries ☐ YES ☐ NO
	Person Reporting:	Position	Local	Critical Incident? ☐ YES ☐ NO
INVESTIGATION INFORMATION	Date Notified (D/M/Y) / /	Time Notified (0000) HOURS	Time on Site (0000) HOURS	INVESTIGATOR(S) _____
	Original BME Contact	Patient Admission #	Physician	_____
INITIAL INCIDENT INFORMATION				

INITIAL INVESTIGATION

1. Initial Observations

A.	BME Notified Immediately	YES ☐	NO ☐
B.	Incident Report Form Completed	YES ☐	NO ☐
C.	Person Reporting Incident Available for Interview	YES ☐	NO ☐
D.	Equipment Is Undisturbed	YES ☐	NO ☐
E.	Accessories Have been Saved	YES ☐	NO ☐

2. Equipment/Accessories Inventory and Condition.   (Insp. Forms Attached: YES☐ NO☐)

Item	Equipment Descriptions and Condition. (Settings?)	Serial, ECN, Lot

3. Description of Patient/ Staff Injuries (Patient Examined by Investigator: YES ☐   NO ☐)
Source of Information: Incident Report☐ Physician☐ Nurse☐ Pt. Record☐ Other☐ _____

_____
_____
_____
_____

4. Initial Incident Findings _____
_____
_____
_____
_____
_____
_____
_____

(Printed with permission from the Biomedical Engineering Department, Vancouver General Hospital)

FOLLOW UP INVESTIGATION

5. Inspections and tests performed on Equipment

Item	Description of tests	Test results

6. Disposable items that have been saved

_____

_____

_____

_____

_____

_____

7. Subsequent investigation results

_____

_____

_____

_____

_____

_____

_____

_____

_____

_____

_____

_____

_____

_____

_____

_____

_____

_____

_____

_____

_____

_____

_____

(Printed with permission from the Biomedical Engineering Department, Vancouver General Hospital)

8. Recommended remedial action

_____
_____
_____
_____
_____
_____
_____
_____
_____
_____
_____
_____
_____
_____
_____
_____
_____
_____
_____

9. Additional comments

_____
_____
_____
_____
_____
_____
_____
_____

10. Documents attached to report

	Type of form	Description	
1.	Incident Investigation Results Letter		YES ☐ NO ☐
2.	Patient / Visitor Incident Report Form		YES ☐ **NO** ☐
3.	Incident Diagrams / Photographs:		YES ☐ NO ☐
4.	Outside Agency & Company Reports		YES ☐ NO ☐
5.	All Correspondence: (list)		YES ☐ NO ☐
6.	Equipment Inspection Forms: (list)		YES ☐ NO ☐
7.	Others:		

Primary Investigator's Signature: _____ Title: _____ Date: _____

Assisting Investigator's Signature: _____ Title: _____ Date: _____

Director's Approval: _____ Date: _____

(Printed with permission from the Biomedical Engineering Department, Vancouver General Hospital)

Chapter 7

INTRODUCTION TO NEEDS ASSESSMENT AND TECHNOLOGY ACQUISITION

Now that we have gained more understanding in the concept of technology management and the technology life cycle, it is now proper to examine in more detail how diffused technologies find their way into clinical use. This chapter focuses on facility-level technology acquisition, which out of necessity includes technology needs assessment. Although most of the discussions are focussed on hospital medical devices, a similar approach can be extended to health technology in general.

1 HOSPITAL-LEVEL TECHNOLOGY ASSESSMENT AND ACQUISITION

The health care system today is facing increasing demands for services while experiencing pressure from upward spiraling costs. As technology has a tremendous impact on the cost and structure of health care delivery, health care facilities need to include technology assessment in both their near and long-term facility planning processes. The assessment and evaluation of health care technologies is a potentially complicated and lengthy process, requiring a multidepartmental approach.

1.1 Assessment Versus Acquisition

Cost-benefit and cost-effectiveness analyses are two of the more common approaches in the economic assessment of medical technologies. Cost-benefit analysis calculates the costs of applying the technology and compares the benefits resulting from its application. It provides a straightforward rule to decide whether to adopt or reject a technology. The technology is adopted if the sum of benefits is greater than the sum of the costs. However, the limitation of this analysis is that all benefits including therapeutic effects have to be expressed in monetary terms. In contrast, cost-effectiveness analysis quantifies therapeutic effects in such terms as reduced hospital-length-of-stay or quality-adjusted-years-of-life-saved and compares them to the costs of technology implementation. However, this approach does not produce explicit decision rules for policy makers such as health insurance agencies.

In medical technology assessment, not only does the process need to identify technologies that improve cost-effectiveness and benefit patient care outcomes, the process needs to include an evaluation scheme so that requests for new technologies competing for common resources may be objectively compared and contrasted. These goals are achievable only when a proactive systematic medical technology assessment and acquisition program has been established. Such a program is to ensure that the decisions to purchase new technologies are based upon careful analysis of reliable and objective data.

The concept of technology assessment is often confused with the concept of technology acquisition. Whereas technology acquisition encompasses the mechanics of the purchasing process, technology assessment is a necessary predecessor of technology acquisition. Technology acquisition includes the following four main processes which are the subject of discussion in the next chapter:

1. budgeting–to estimate all costs associated with the acquisition and deployment of the technology
2. tender preparation and tendering
3. selection–which includes technical and clinical evaluations as well as financial analysis
4. award of contract

Technology assessment evaluates the technology according to four different criteria, including:

1. the technology's feasibility, that it, the technology's technical ability to actually accomplish its stated conceptual goal or objective
2. the technology's efficacy, that is, the ability of the technology to accomplish its goal or objective under ideal conditions
3. the technology's effectiveness, or its ability to accomplish its goal or objective under nonideal clinical conditions
4. the technology's economic benefit, that is, the technology's cost effectiveness and cost benefit

1.2 Scope of Hospital-Level Technology Assessment

Not only is it important to establish a technology's ability to accomplish its stated goals or objectives at the clinical level, it is necessary to understand the impact of the technology on all levels of the facility, as well as for the greater community. The needs of each individual facility vary depending on the characteristics of institutions. For example, a research-based facility may be involved in all the above four criteria. For the most part, general hospitals are more concerned with purchases of proven technologies which should fulfill a need in the facility (e.g., clinical requirement, safety, etc.) or provide some benefits (e.g., reduce operating costs, reduce patient-length-of-stay, etc.); that is, primarily item four and perhaps some of item three of the above criteria. In all cases, a strategic technology planning and assessment process will lead to improved cost-efficiency and overall patient health care.

The topic of technology assessment has been and continues to be the focus of much work and studies. To limit the scope, the discussion of technology assessment in this book is curtailed to hospital-level technology assessment. That is, it will focus on cost-effectiveness and cost-benefit analysis. The first three technology assessment criteria will only be covered briefly. Even in this very limited scope, the concept of hospital level technology assessment and planning is still very broad and includes the following facets:

- *Identifying technologies that complement existing services.* Through the strategic planning process, the services provided by the facility are first identified. Often, the technologies required to deliver and support these services will naturally surface thereafter.

- *Analyzing the effects of new equipment on existing services.* While the chosen technology may appear at first glance to have little impact on other facility operations, it is important that all potential impact are identified, especially in the environmental and operational aspects.

- *Evaluation of productivity and quality of patient care.* Assessing current technologies to identify instances in which new technology may affect productivity and quality of patient care (such as patient length of stay, device downtime, supply costs, etc.) is one of the most important considerations of the technology planning process. Coupled with this is the aspect of identifying potential hazardous technology that needs to be replaced.

- *Assessment of long-term replacement strategies.* One of the most common assumptions and often-overlooked aspect of technology planning is the development of a long-range technology replacement plan. Very few technologies and almost zero medical devices have infinite longevity. No measure of preventive maintenance will keep devices working forever, so it is best to plan well ahead in order to minimize the impact of unexpected large-ticket capital replacement.

- *Identifying emerging technologies.* A proactive and somewhat predictive approach to technology planning is essential in areas where population demographics, environmental conditions, and other factors can lead to major changes in health care requirements. By identifying emerging technologies that fit into the projected demographics of the facility's service area, a facility may avoid bad investment decisions and reduce unnecessary expenditures (e.g., investing in a near obsolete technology).

Technology planning strategy based on the results from sound technology assessment will provide better investment returns and significantly improve patient outcomes.

2 INFRASTRUCTURE REQUIREMENTS

Perhaps the key infrastructure component required for successful implementation of a systematic technology assessment and acquisition process is the establishment of a group of competent individuals to oversee and manage the process. For the purpose of our discussion, this group will be referred to as the Capital Equipment Review Committee (CERC). Of equal importance is to establish a number of working groups to carry out the necessary functions to acquire the technology. For our discussion, we refer to them as the Technology Acquisition Working Groups (TAWG). Control of the overall capital budget typically remains the responsibility of a Capital Budget Committee (CBC). The CBC usually consists of senior facility administrators and/or board members.

2.1 Capital Equipment Review Committee (CERC)

The primary purpose of the CERC is to coordinate the overall capital equipment assessment and acquisition process from a hospital-wide perspective based upon both clinical and administrative requirements. As such, the CERC must:
- gather and analyze operational plans from the administrative to the departmental level
- collect and analyze technology information such as existing medical device inventory and capital requests
- ultimately use this information to create a comprehensive and justifiable equipment procurement and assets management plan

It must be noted that it is not usually the mandate of the CERC to generate or initiate the equipment acquisition process. However, the CERC may in the course of its activities initiate some. The process of initiating equipment acquisition lies predominantly with the users, e.g., medical staff in the clinical department. The primary responsibility of the CERC is to evaluate and assess these capital equipment requests. With a facility-wide perspective, the CERC will submit to the CBC (Capital Budget Committee) a prioritized list of suggested capital equipment acquisitions for the current fiscal year, as well as informing them of future equipment needs. In smaller facilities, a combined capital committee may fulfill the roles of both the CERC and CBC. The process and sequence of analyzing capital requests by the CERC will be studied in more details later in this chapter.

The CERC performs its duty by considering both the clinical and administrative perspectives of the facility while taking into consideration the limited hospital-wide capital funding available. The CERC establishes the priority based on factual information such as needs, benefits, and costs. For this reason, membership of the CERC must be composed of personnel with both clinical and administrative backgrounds as well as with technical and financial knowledge. Figure 7–1 shows the composition of a typical CERC. Notice that the membership includes both users and supporting services. Since the CERC is a working committee, its membership is not restricted to those members identified in the example (Fig. 7–1). Occasionally the CERC may recruit temporary members with complementary skills from clinical, administrative, or technical areas, especially when special technical or medical questions are encountered.

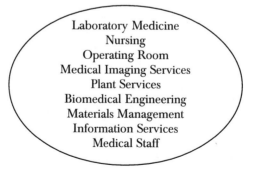

Laboratory Medicine
Nursing
Operating Room
Medical Imaging Services
Plant Services
Biomedical Engineering
Materials Management
Information Services
Medical Staff

Figure 7–1. CERC Membership Composition.

2.2 Technology Acquisition Working Group (TAWG)

The function of the Technology Acquisition Working Group (TAWG) is to carry out the work for acquiring the technology. Usually, the TAWG performs its duties by utilizing the expertise of the in-house users and support staff. Occasionally, outside help may be sought. Its activities include defining and evaluating the clinical and support requirements and analyzing the financial implications of the technology. The tasks may include:

- Prepare general and functional specifications
- Come up with a short list of vendors
- Analyze tender proposals
- Conduct clinical and technical evaluations
- Perform cost analysis
- Review evaluation results
- Negotiate and finalize details of the purchase contract

Usually, the TAWG is a working team which is formed when the technology acquisition is approved by the CBC and will be dissolved when the purchase contract (or purchase order) is issued. Depending on the nature of the technology to be acquired, the team usually consists of representatives from the clinical user departments, the purchasing department, as well as from the support and servicing areas. Figure 7–2 gives an example of the composition of a team for the acquisition of a video endoscopic system in the outpatient endoscopy suite of a hospital.

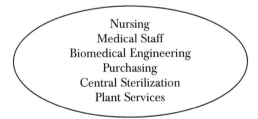

Nursing
Medical Staff
Biomedical Engineering
Purchasing
Central Sterilization
Plant Services

Figure 7–2. TAWG Membership Composition for Video Endoscopy Acquisition.

3 NEEDS IDENTIFICATION

One of the initial tasks that must be done in the assessment and acquisition process is to define the clinical needs. Needs identification usually starts from the users of the technology such as medical staff or nurses. Allied health professionals (such as biomedical engineers, respiratory therapists) or support services groups (such as central sterilization department, physical plant) may participate and often facilitate the process. The needs to acquire a technology may be one or a combination of the following:

- to provide needed service
- to improve service efficiency
- to improve clinical outcomes
- to increases cost effectiveness or cost benefit
- to meet minimum standards
- to reduce risk
- to cope with change patient characteristics in the primary referral base

The next task is to outline the scope of the clinical requirements based on the identified needs. This is performed through input from multiple professional groups or individuals upon whom the new technology will have impact, such as physicians, medical lab technologists, and support services. While the individual or group requesting the technology provides much of the required information, additional research must be performed at this time to identify what devices or systems are available, what are the key desirable features and functions, etc. This review process may be as easy as an informal market survey and literature search or it may require establishing an investigation committee to conduct extensive data collection and analysis. While this review is in progress, a list of possible vendors should also be developed.

One of the more difficult tasks in needs identification is to differentiate the "must have" features from the "nice to have" features. A list of all these features and accessories should be maintained for discussion and review by the TAWG before the final purchase.

The development of clinical requirement specifications allows the facility to precisely and succinctly define goals and clinical objectives of the technology as they relate to the situation at hand. As mentioned earlier, this is not a "wish-list," but a "must-have" list. Establishing these requirements at an early stage will help to focus the assessment and acquisition process, and will allow the requesting department to be certain of what is or what is not to be purchased.

4 THE FACILITY-LEVEL TECHNOLOGY ACQUISITION PROCESS

Generally speaking, the acquisition of technology in a health care facility can be subdivided into four phases.

1. Identifying needs and defining clinical requirements by the users of the technology. This is followed by the development of specifications based on the identified needs and clinical requirements, as well as other nonfunctional needs related to the technology such as in-service education, repair, and preventive maintenance.
2. Execution of tendering procedures incorporating the specifications and the facility's financial planning activities.
3. Analysis, evaluations, and decision making based on the technical, clinical, and financial perspectives.
4. Preparing and awarding the purchase order or contract.

A flowchart showing the tasks and information flow in a comprehensive technology acquisition process is shown in Figure 7–3. Dialogues established between all involved parties are essential to ensure that the most appropriate technology is being acquired and that all possible issues have been addressed, including standardization, costs of installation, maintenance, optimal use of funds, etc. Certain aspects of this process will be discussed in more detail in the next chapter.

Health care facilities need to establish a formal review process that allows a qualitative and quantitative evaluation of the needs for the technology in the facility. This process usually involves a variety of different departments in the facility, as it is a multidepartmental process. For large-ticket items, the review may require a major technology assessment. For less-expensive and "every-day" type items (including replacement items), this review may simply consist of a review of the current needs of the department and the operational and financial impact of the new equipment.

As mentioned in the previous section, it is typically the case that physicians and medical personnel initiate new or replacement equipment requests. However, proactive technology planning can also have these initiatives taken place through a number of alternative sources. For example, it is more economical for a facility to replace an older device which requires excessive maintenance costs (such as an old x-

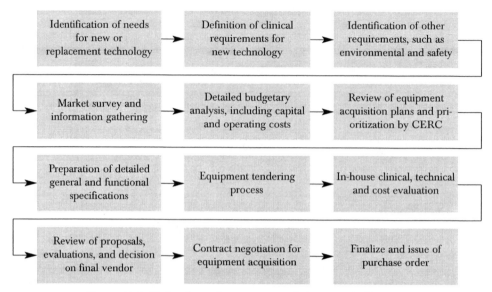

Figure 7–3. Technology Assessment and Acquisition Process.

ray machine which needs frequent tube replacement). In another case, it makes sense to replace old equipment with a new one that uses substantially less expensive consumables. In both of the above-mentioned situations, the initiation of the technology assessment and acquisition process would more appropriately stem from the in-house biomedical engineering department or someone responsible for maintaining the device who maintains an awareness of new technological trends and development.

4.1 Department Equipment Acquisition Plan (DEAP)

Generally speaking, it is the responsibility of each department or cost center to develop and maintain a multiple-year, capital equipment replacement plan for the department. Such a Department Equipment Acquisition Plan (DEAP) will be submitted to the CERC at the beginning of the capital acquisition cycle. A DEAP is a capital equipment request list; each item in the plan should contain the following information:

- Device description
- Quantity requested
- Estimated cost (including supplies and installation)

- Whether it is a new or replacement unit. The age of the old equipment.
- A brief justification of the requisition
- The priority rank among the items in the plan

The CERC will review and consolidate all DEAP's to maintain an overall multiple year (e.g., three-year) acquisition plan for the facility. Once all individual requests have been reviewed and prioritized for the entire hospital, the capital acquisition plan for the current fiscal year is submitted to the CBC for final approval and budget allocation. The details of this process will be discussed in greater depth later in the chapter. The entire process is greatly enhanced through the use of a computerized system, which automatically tracks the individual requests, or even performs automatic prioritization once the required information is supplied.

4.2 Proposal for Capital Equipment Acquisition (PCEA)

The primary purpose of the DEAP is to aid the CERC and hospital administration in both short- and long-range technology acquisition planning; each item in the DEAP should be accompanied by a Proposal for Capital Equipment Acquisition (PCEA) which states the rationales for the acquisition request. The PCEA submissions are reviewed and assessed by the CERC to generate the facility-wide capital acquisition plan.

In practice, it is not uncommon to have different PCEA forms for different categories of equipment. It is certainly beneficial to use different forms for equipment of different price ranges, as opposed to one form for all. The rationale arises from the point of view of cost benefit consideration, the amount of information and the process of completing and evaluating a PCEA for an inexpensive item should be less and simpler than those for an expensive one.

PCEA forms are designed to facilitate detailed analysis of the proposed equipment acquisition. As the cost of the requested equipment increases, the CERC will need more information to justify the prioritization decision. Obviously, a request for a $1 million diagnostic system should be more closely scrutinized than a request for a $2000 microscope. It is also desirable to have different PCEA forms for medical and nonmedical devices, as this will ensure capital requests are evaluated against relevant items in the same category. A sample copy of a PCEA (Fig. 7–4) is appended to the end of this chapter. Furthermore, it is important that the evaluation criteria for capital acquisition are defined to ensure that sufficient technical evaluation and cost analysis are performed, especially for emerging technologies.

5. POTENTIAL PROBLEMS WITH ACQUISITION PROCESSES

With increasing equipment sophistication, escalating operating costs, and overwhelming number of options, it is essential to have a systematic and comprehensive technology acquisition program in place in order to prevent a number of potential problems associated with technology acquisition. Some of these problems may arise from the following situations:

5.1 Lack of Hospital-wide Capital Process

Many hospitals do not have a hospital-wide process to prioritize capital requests. Some hospitals may arbitrarily divide the capital budget among the clinical areas without a systematic evaluation process. The priority of an individual equipment request must be ascertained by reviewing a number of issues such as strategic, clinical, fiscal, and operational. Without a thorough facility-wide review, it is not possible to rationally determine which equipment should be purchased in lieu of another request. Ideally, equipment with the greatest net positive impact should be purchased, but this may not be obvious without going through a thorough assessment process. This problem is obvious when departments are allocated fixed capital equipment budgets. In some years, a department may not be able to acquire much needed equipment. In other years, the same departments may have funds to purchase equipment which is of lower priority than those requested by other departments.

5.2 Technology Being Used in Multiple Areas

It was discussed earlier that allowing too many makes and models of a device to be used in a hospital has many disadvantages. In a hospital, it is desirable to have as few makes and models of the same type of medical device as possible. Medical device and product standardization can be achieved by proper coordination of equipment acquisition activities. Although capital acquisitions that involve many user groups are difficult to coordinate (as different users tend to have their own preferences and subjective opinions), dispute can be avoided by clearly identifying the needs and defining the evaluation criteria early in the process.

5.3 Failure to Perform Impact Studies

The impact of the technology to the facility (especially if it is new to the facility) must be carefully and completely considered before it is purchased. The entire life cycle of the equipment must be considered, including initial purchase cost, installation cost, staffing requirements, operating cost, maintenance cost, etc. For larger-ticket items, these costs must be weighed against the benefits to the hospital and the community as a whole, and may involve the need for a thorough cost-benefit analysis.

5.4 Inadequate Equipment Replacement and Acquisition Planning

Occasionally, it is possible that, by replacing obsolete or older equipment, the facility could obtain overall savings by proactively replacing equipment before it is found to be irreparable or no longer clinically acceptable. As well, many requests for equipment replacement may be planned well in advance of the actual date of replacement. Equipment replacement planning provides these benefits if it can be effectively done both at the departmental level and on a facility-wide basis. Multiple years planning for expensive items can soften the impact on the annual capital budget. This subject will be considered in more detail in the next chapter.

5.5 Other Problems

In addition to the above, there are other problems related to this topic. Examples include duplication of requests by two departments, tendency to assign a lower priority to nonmedical equipment requests, inappropriate use of senior administrators' time in assessing capital requests, etc.

6 A SYSTEMATIC ACQUISITION PROCESS

It is essential to systematize, formalize, and document the assessment and acquisition process in today's highly complex medical facilities. It is only with such a system approach that all aspects of the technology's life cycle can be considered and adequately addressed. A system approach will reveal hidden costs associated with the technology before making the final decision.

When considering the actual capital costs of a new technology, medical staffs often overlook the needs for enabling capital expenditures. These expenditures include items such as major renovation (e.g., structural reinforcement for heavy equipment), user education (including both operation and service training), and the needs to special utilities (e.g., plumbing and gas, air conditioning, electricity, etc.).

The purchase of a new technology must be justified by an increase in equipment cost-effectiveness. The following questions should be asked when performing the analysis:
- Will it increase the volume of service?
- Will there be an increase in the overall cost of the service?
- Will it expand an existing service?
- Will it provide a new revenue-generating service?

In order to demonstrate cost-effectiveness over time, the life cycle costs and benefits must be reviewed. Questions asked during such analysis may include:
- What is the expected life span of the new technology?
- What impact does the technology have on operating costs, such as disposables, utilities, and staffing?
- Will there be an increase in departmental efficiency if this equipment is purchased?
- What is the expected annual workload volume for this equipment over the life span of the technology?
- What will be the cost of disposal?

Since operating costs can be as high and even higher than the initial capital cost, it is important to address these questions before a new technology is acquired. A detailed cost-benefit/cost-effectiveness analysis will provide answers to these questions. Such analysis should, at a minimum, take into account the costs of human resources, space, utilities (power, air, gas, water, waste, housekeeping, environmental factors, etc.), and the end-of-use disposal costs.

In order to assess the benefit of a technology, some key patient-care outcome indicators must be reviewed. For example, the analysis would factor in the cost saving of moving the patient from the intensive care ward to a general patient care area or explore the potential to reduce length-of-stay of patients in the hospital. In addition, there are many other nonquantitative outcomes that must be evaluated when considering a new technology. Even though a detailed discussion of the quality of life is beyond the scope of this book, it should be one of the important considerations.

Another reason to conduct a formal review is to ensure that the requested technology will enhance current and future needs of patient care. An obvious example of such needs is patient safety (and of course, the safety of the staff using the technology). Questions to be asked in the area of patient safety may include:

- Are there safety standard deficiencies that the new technology is designed to address?
- Are there hospital accreditation standards or operational standards that the new technology will fulfill?
- When it comes to replacing older technology, will the failure to purchase this new equipment pose a risk to the patients who are presently being treated with this old equipment?
- May the addition of this equipment reduce the risk of injury or occupational hazards among staff members?

7 SOURCES OF INFORMATION

Other than the manufacturers and suppliers, there are many government and private agencies from which one can obtain information in technology planning and acquisitions. Listed below are some of these sources:

- FDA (Food and Drug Administration, http://www.fda.gov/)– U.S. government regulatory agency that regulates and assesses technologies before they are approved for use by the public.
- NIH (National Institute of Health, http://www.nih.gov/)–a U.S. organization supports clinical research in the U.S. and funds technology assessment
- OTA (Office of Technology Assessment–closed in 1995, the site archives all publications, http://www.wws.princeton.edu/~ota/)

- CCOHTA (Canadian Coordinating Office of Health Technology Assessment, http://www.ccohta.ca/)–A Canadian government-funded organization to provide evidence-based information on emerging and existing health technologies, primarily to Canadian health care policy makers and managers.
- BCOHTA (The British Columbia Office of Health Technology Assessment, http://www.chspr.ubc.ca/)–A B.C. Provincial Government funded organization which promotes and encourages the use of health technology assessment research, appropriate to issues of policy, planning, and utilization at governmental, operational, and clinical levels.
- ECRI (formally known as the Emergency Care Research Institute, http://healthcare.ecri.org/)–an independent nonprofit health services research agency in the U.S.
- INAHTA (International Network of Agencies for Health Technology Assessment, http://www.inahta.org/)
- ISTAHC (International Society of Technology Assessment in Health Care, http://www.istahc.org/)

Figure 7–4.

Example of
PROPOSAL FOR CAPITAL EQUIPMENT ACQUISITION (PCEA)

MEDICAL EQUIPMENT (Purchase price greater than $100,000)

PCEA No. _____ Date Requested: _____ Priority: _____

DIVISION/DEPARTMENT: _____ DATE: _____

CONTACT PERSON: _____ PHONE: _____

DEVICE DESCRIPTION: _____

REPLACEMENT OR NEW

NUMBER REQUIRED: _____ TOTAL COST:$ _____

A. DESCRIPTION OF EQUIPMENT

1.0 *GENERAL DESCRIPTION*

1.1 Briefly describe the function and purpose of the equipment? If this equipment is part of a larger system, describe the system.

1.2 How will the new equipment be cost-effective, e.g., will it increase volume of service at the same cost? Show any evidence of volume increases for your service. Please specify.

2.0 *PURPOSE OF REQUEST*

2.1 Discuss in detail what the exact purpose of this equipment in your department will be, i.e., why the equipment is required.

2.2 Has this equipment been requested to
i) expand existing service?
     YES _____ NO _____
ii) provide a new service?
     YES _____ NO _____
ii) other? Please specify.

2.3 How is this particular service currently being handled in the hospital? In the community?

2.4 Does the requested item meet existing patient care needs?
     YES _____ NO _____ N/A _____
Explain how the item enhances patient care.

How does the requested item meet future patient care needs?

2.5 Is this equipment being requested to meet established
     i) Safety standards?   YES _____ NO _____
     ii) Hospital accreditation standards?   YES _____ NO _____
     iii) Department accreditation standards?   YES _____ NO _____
     iv) CSA standards?   YES _____ NO _____
     If YES, please specify.

2.6 May the failure to purchase this equipment pose a risk to the safety of patients who are
     presently being treated without this equipment?
              YES _____ NO _____ N/A _____
     If YES, please specify.

2.7 May the addition of this equipment reduce risk of injury or occupational disease in the
     staff who will be treating the patients?
              YES _____ NO _____ N/A _____
     If YES, please specify.

3.0 *SPECIFIC DESCRIPTION OF MANUFACTURER*
3.1 Who is the proposed manufacturer? What is the requested equipment item, i.e., model
     number, accessories, and options? How many are requested?

3.2 Has this equipment been evaluated in your department?
              YES _____ NO _____

3.3 Can this equipment and/or system be upgraded or expanded to meet increases in depart-
     ment workload or changing patient needs?
              YES _____ NO _____ N/A _____
     If YES, list upgrade, its cost, the reason for acquiring it, and the approximate time-frame
     for its purchase.

3.4 What is the proposed life of the equipment?
              <3 yrs _____ <5 yrs _____ <10 yrs _____ >10 yrs _____

3.5 Describe the warranty and available maintenance contracts that are offered by the com-
     pany. What is covered under these (i.e., parts, labor, etc.)?

Who is to perform the following tasks:
i) preventive maintenance?
manufacturer _____ in-house _____ other _____
ii) service maintenance (i.e., repair)?
manufacturer _____ in-house _____ other _____

3.6 Are there other manufactures with similar equipment?
YES _____ NO _____
Have these been considered?
YES _____ NO _____

4.0 *REPLACEMENT (if applicable)*
4.1 Describe the item that is being replaced.

What is the age of this item?
<3 yrs _____ <5 yrs _____ <10 yrs _____ >10 yrs _____

4.2 Is the old equipment obsolete? Why? Be specific.

B. STRATEGIC GOALS OF HOSPITAL
1.0 *STRATEGIC GOALS*
1.1 Discuss how this equipment purchase coincides with established short- and long-term goals and strategies of:
i) the department.

ii) the hospital.

iii) the Ministry of Health.

C. IMPACT OF THIS EQUIPMENT ON THE HOSPITAL
1.0 *IMPACT ON SERVICES*
1.1 Is there potential for collaborating with other facilities for sharing the requested equipment? What would the arrangements be? Is the other department in agreement?

2.0 *IMPACT ON RESOURCES*
2.1 What is the impact of this equipment on departmental operations in terms of staffing, maintenance, etc.?

2.2 Will there be an increase in departmental efficiency if this equipment is purchased?

YES _____ NO _____ N/A _____

If YES, explain the reasons for this increase in efficiency.

2.3 What is the expected annual workload volumes for this equipment over the next five years?

	Year 1	Year 2	Year 3	Year 4	Year 5
INPATIENT					
OUTPATIENT					

3.4 Include any other comments in support of this submission.

D. SITE PLANNING AND INFORMATION

1. Where is this equipment to be used?

2. Is there a need for any building modifications, i.e., plumbing and gas considerations, air conditioning, electrical?

YES _____ NO _____ N/A _____

If YES, please give details.

3. Are there requirements for

i) detailed site planning?   YES _____ NO _____
ii installation schedule?   YES _____ NO _____
iii) acceptance inspection documentation?   YES _____ NO _____

If YES, please elaborate on who is to provide these and briefly explain these requirements.

4. Is there need for a patient waiting room and/or large item supply storage?

YES _____ NO _____

Has ample room been set aside for such in your current facilities?

YES _____ NO _____

E. TRAINING AND STAFF QUALIFICATIONS

1. Does the department's staff have the qualifications necessary to operate this equipment?

YES _____ NO _____

Does the department require additional qualified personnel?

YES _____ NO _____

If YES, explain how this additional staffing requirement will be met.

2. Have appropriate staff qualifications been recommended by the manufacturer?
    YES _____ NO _____

3. Is there a need for operational staff training?
    YES _____ NO _____
    If YES:
    Is this to be provided by the
    i) manufacturer?   YES _____ NO _____
    ii) in-house?   YES _____ NO _____
    iii) other?   YES _____ NO _____
    Have the time and location of this training been arranged?
    YES _____ NO _____

4. Who will provide in-servicing for this equipment?
    i) manufacturer?   YES _____ NO _____
    ii) in-house?   YES _____ NO _____
    iii) other?   YES _____ NO _____

F. COST ANALYSIS
1.0 *START-UP COSTS AND BENEFITS*

1.1 For this equipment, what is the total purchase price?
    i) purchase cost? $ _____
    ii) applicable taxes? $ _____
    iii) shipping charges? $ _____
    iv) custom charges? $ _____

    TOTAL PURCHASE PRICE $ _____

1.2 What are the set-up costs?
    i) capital renovations? $ _____
    ii) installation? $ _____
    iii) staff training? $ _____

    TOTAL SET-UP COST $ _____

Have capital renovation costs been:
    i) budgeted?   YES _____ NO _____
    ii) approved?   YES _____ NO _____
Have installation costs been:
    i) budgeted?   YES _____ NO _____
    ii) approved?   YES _____ NO _____
Have staff training costs been:
    i) budgeted?   YES _____ NO _____
    ii) approved?   YES _____ NO _____

1.3 Is any capital funding available from:
    i) trade-in allowance? YES _____ NO _____
        If YES, specify amount. $ _____
    ii) resale value?   YES _____ NO _____
        If YES, specify amount. $ _____
    Specify to whom it could be sold?

2.0 *ANNUAL COSTS AND BENEFITS*

2.1 What are the additional annual operating costs (savings) over five years, including the costs of contract maintenance, preventive maintenance, operating supplies, additional staff, possible repair costs, any hardware and firmware updates, utilities, and insurance?
    Have maintenance costs been:
        i) budgeted?   YES _____ NO _____
        ii) approved?   YES _____ NO _____
    Have operating supplies costs been:
        i) budgeted?   YES _____ NO _____
        ii) approved?   YES _____ NO _____
    Have additional staffing costs been:
        i) budgeted?   YES _____ NO _____
        ii) approved?   YES _____ NO _____

    Please complete summary table.

SUMMARY CHART

	YEAR 1	YEAR 2	YEAR 3	YEAR 4	YEAR 5
REVENUE Ministry of Health: Research: Donations: Other:					

COSTS
Start-up:
Operational:
  supplies
  extra staff
  utilities
  insurance
Maintenance:
  contract
  other					

Chapter 8

BUDGETING

Budgeting is the first step in hospital level technology acquisition. A detailed consideration of all possible expenditures throughout the life cycle of the technology will provide critical information in technology planning and acquisition. It will avoid surprises and ensure a smooth deployment of the technology.

1 COST OF OWNERSHIP

When one considers acquiring a new medical technology, it is very common to focus only on the acquisition cost. However, in many cases, other costs associated with the technology far exceed the acquisition cost. The acquisition cost instead may just be the tip of the iceberg, as shown in Figure 8–1.

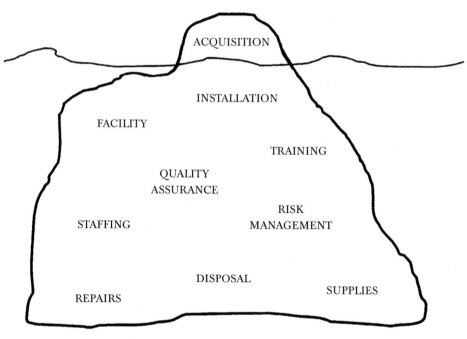

Figure 8–1. Overall Cost of a Technology.

The health facility should consider all costs incurred throughout the entire life of the technology. The cost of ownership or the overall life-cycle cost of a technology should include capital costs, operating expenditures, and disposal costs. Capital and disposal are often one-time costs whereas operating costs are recurring.

2 CAPITAL COSTS

Capital costs are the initial expenditure to acquire and to set up the technology before it can be used. It general, capital costs include:

2.1 Acquisition Cost

This is the cost to acquire the actual equipment including hardware and software and the necessary accessories. For example, a full body multi-slice computer tomography (CT) scanner may cost $900,000 and a laser camera to create hard copies of the CT images may cost another $60,000. To interface it with the existing PACS (Picture Archiving and Communication System) and the RIS (Radiation Information System) may cost another $80,000.

2.2 Installation and Set-up Cost

Some technology may require substantial installation and set-up. For example, to install and set up a magnetic resonance imaging (MRI) scanner will require shipment and delivery of the MRI to the hospital, transporting the unit from the loading dock to the MRI room (which may involve building temporary access for the bulky components), renovation which includes construction of the foundation and installation of the room magnetic shielding, cable connections to the PACS (picture archiving and communication system) and RIS (radiology information system), commissioning, etc.

3 OPERATING EXPENDITURES

Operating expenditures include expenses to support the safe and effective ongoing use of the technology. Operating expenditures may include:

3.1 Facility Cost

This includes the cost of space and utilities such as electricity, water, gases, etc. For some facilities space may not be an issue, but for many, the space occupied can instead generate revenue (e.g., it can be rented out as a gift shop).

3.2 Supplies Cost

Most technology will require operating consumables or disposables. For example, one infusion pump may require 200 disposable infusion sets per year. If each one costs $5 and the hospital has 200 pumps, the annual cost of IV sets totals to $200,000. An X-ray machine needs films and processing chemicals as well as periodic X-ray tube replacements. All of which are cost items.

3.3 Staffing Cost

When evaluating technology, staffing requirement is an important factor, as it will directly affect the cost to run the technology and also affect the efficiency of operation of the technology. The skill level and the number of staff needed to operate the equipment and to care for the patients should be identified and factored into the cost of ownership.

3.4 Training Cost

Some technology requires costly initial training and refresher training. The costs of users and support staff training should be included in the life-cycle expenses of the technology. The cost of service training to maintenance staff is often ignored in the capital tendering process. Without adequate in-house support, hospitals often end up with expensive external service contracts after the equipment warranty has expired.

3.5 Maintenance and Repair Cost

Maintenance and repair can be an expensive cost item over the life-time of a technology. An annual service contract can cost between 5 to 15 percent of the acquisition cost. In addition, frequent breakdowns and lengthy preventive maintenance procedures can create loss of revenue due to unavailability of the equipment.

3.6 Quality Assurance Cost

In addition to performing routine PM inspections to ensure proper performance of the technology, some medical devices or systems require special functional tests and calibration at more frequent intervals. Running QA tests every day on a blood gas analyzer in the medical laboratory, which includes labor and reagents, is an example of such quality assurance cost.

3.7 Risk Management Cost

Apart from the expense for general risk management activities, unreliable medical technology may expose the hospital to liability litigation. Most health care facilities purchase liability insurance to cover the risk that may arise from misuse or failure of technology.

4 DISPOSAL COSTS

The costs of disposal includes the disposal of consumables and the removal and disposal of equipment:

4.1 Disposal of Consumables

Some procedures may create hazardous waste that will require special disposal procedures. For example, in many countries, human specimens and items such as epidemic needles are considered as biological hazardous waste and need to be incinerated at high temperature in special incinerators.

4.2 Disposal of Equipment

When a piece of equipment is being retired, the facility may be able to recover some value from selling the equipment. On the other hand, it may cost the facility to dismantle, remove, and dispose of the equipment. Equipment disposal is discussed in more detail in the next chapter.

5 OTHER IMPACTS

Deploying a new technology may impact other areas of the hospital. Such impact may include human resources, policies and procedures, facilities, equipment, and supplies. For example, when a hospital introduces a fast-acting anesthetic agent to decrease the patients' stay in the operating room to increase OR throughput, it will affect the patient flow pattern in the operating room (OR), the post anesthesia recovery (PAR), and other areas in the hospital. Such impacts and cost evaluation should be considered at the technology assessment phase.

6 LEASING, RENTAL AND PAY-PER-USE

6.1 Leasing versus Purchasing

Some vendors may offer an option to lease rather than to purchase the technology. A health care facility can lease a technology from a private company by paying a monthly leasing fee. Usually, a lease contract will include preventive maintenance and repair costs. Some may even include consumables. The health care facility will then only be responsible for other operating expenses. The advantages of leasing for a health care facility in general are listed below:
- No up-front lump sum capital cost. The money may then be invested in other areas to generate revenue.
- No additional cost on repair and maintenance (if they are included in the lease agreement).
- No worry about technology obsolescence.

The disadvantages of leasing for the facility are:
- No ownership of the equipment.
- No scavenged value of the equipment at the end of the lease.
- Greater cost to lease than to buy.

To determine whether to lease or to purchase, one will have to weigh the advantages of leasing against the cost of leasing. The cost analysis requires comparing the net present values of the life-cycle cost between the two (net present value analysis will be covered later in this chapter).

6.2 Rental

Oftentimes, medical devices are underutilized in health care facilities. For example, 100 infusion pumps may be procured by a hospital to meet the peak demand, while in most days, only 60 are required. Purchase (or lease) only makes sense when devices are under high utilization. An alternative is medical device rental (sometimes refers to by some vendors as fleet management). Health care facilities can assess their weekly or even daily requirements and rent devices to meet the immediate needs. For the infusion pump example mentioned above, the hospital can reach an agreement with a fleet management company to have 60 pumps on site for a fixed rental fee while keeping track of the demand fluctuation daily and order more at a predetermined rate when needed. Most vendors providing such services will guarantee same-day delivery. Rental devices are usually on high volume items such as infusion pumps and oxygen concentrators. The advantages of this strategy include those of leasing listed above plus the following:

- Increase medical device utilization (i.e., less idling equipment).
- No commitment to pay for a fixed number of devices for a fixed period of time.
- Devices can be ordered on demand.
- Less storage space required (no more idling equipment occupying floor space).

6.3 Pay-Per-Use

Although it is not yet very popular, a variation of rental is "pay-per-use." The idea of this strategy is similar to rental except that the rent is based on the number of times the device is actually used instead of on a daily or weekly basis. For example, a hospital has installed a point-of-care blood gas analyzer in the intensive care unit. Instead of being charged for a fixed rental fee, the hospital is charged for the number of blood gas examinations performed at an agreed rate. A pay-per-use approach provides a direct method to account for the cost of services used by the patients, especially when medical services are rendered on a fee-for-service basis. However, it requires additional means to track and record the types of procedures and the number of times the procedures were performed. In fact, this approach has been used for a long time in medical laboratories where some vendors provide laboratory analyzers free to the hospital and change only the consumables.

6.4 Application Service Providers

This is another variation of pay-per-use. Instead of using this approach on hardware, the vendor provides "soft" services (such as providing application programs or data storage service) to health care facilities. Such vendors are commonly being referred to as "Application Service Providers" or ASP.

An example of ASP service is in PACS (Picture Archiving and Communications System): A medical imaging department in a hospital generates terabytes (a byte is a unit to measure the storage requirement or the amount of information in digital format, a terabyte = 10^{12} bytes) of images every year. A PACS system provides the storage and communication functions for the retrieval, analysis, and transportation functions of the images for radiologists and other physicians. A PACS system requires viewing workstations, computer servers, application software as well as data storage space. The ASP may supply the application software and provide the data bank off site for the hospital to store the images. The hospital is charged on the number of transactions and the data storage capacity. Under this arrangement, the hospital only needs to lease or purchase the workstations and provide the communication links to the ASP's data center.

Noted below is a list of factors in favor of the ASP model from the user's perspective:
- Faster implementation
- Avoid expensive capital expenditures
- No need to worry about technology obsolescence
- Reduce the need for in-house specialists
- Able to access to application specific expertise from the ASP
- Reduce the need for providing training to in-house staff to keep up with the technology
- Predictable cash flow

The main drawback of the ASP model is the continuous reliance on external resources for the service.

Chapter 9

HOSPITAL-LEVEL
TECHNOLOGY ACQUISITION

Once the Capital Budget Committee (CBC) has approved the technology acquisition after reviewing the capital and operational budget, the Technology Acquisition Working Group (TAWG) will begin the tendering process. The tendering process serves the following purposes in technology acquisition:

- It ensures that the product requirements are accurately conveyed to the potential suppliers.
- It allows the vendors to bid under a fair environment.
- It enables the requester to select the best possible device or system.
- It protects the purchasers from not receiving the promised goods and services from the selected vendor.

1 THE TENDERING PROCESS

The tender document translates the needs of the users and the requirements of the facility into a comprehensive document to facilitate a fair bidding process. It will also provide a guide to develop criteria for the evaluation of vendors and their products.

In order to save time and resources, if the technology to be purchased is fairly standard and does not entail major budgetary consideration or complicated interactions with other equipment, then the facility could proceed to purchase the item by requesting vendors to submit quotations on the items requested. However, if it is not a typical purchase, or entails large capital outlay, or has very special requirements, then a more detailed specification, tendering, and bidding process should be carried out. This section will deal primarily with the latter case.

1.1 Specifications

In the process of acquiring medical devices and systems, preparing specifications is the next step following needs definition and preliminary budgeting. Although not all equipment acquisition requires detailed specifications, the benefits in terms of simplifying the tender evaluation based on the specified "need" versus "nice-to-have" features and the time savings from dealing with ambiguities in the tender responses will outweigh the effort put in. Specifications must be carefully written so that selected vendors can submit meaningful proposals. A suggested specification format is as shown on the next page.

Tender Document
Scope
- List of applicable documents
- Precedence and changes

Purpose
- Needs, goals and objectives
- Operational concepts

Requirements
- Objectives
- General requirements
- Specific requirements

Delivery, Tests, Acceptance, and Payment Conditions
- Delivery schedule
- Verification and validation tests
- Acceptance criteria
- Terms of payment

1.1.1 General Specifications

Many requirements in a specification document are common to most medical devices and systems. Compliance with the electrical safety standards is one example. Therefore, a general specification document that applies to most medical device purchases can be developed to save development time and to avoid omissions. A general specification document may include the following information:
- Regulatory and standards compliance
- General installation requirements
- Utilities requirements
- Vendor testing obligations
- Training
- User support
- Warranty
- Maintenance and service support
- Documentation requirements
- Sources of replacement parts
- General evaluation and testing statements

1.1.2 Specific Requirements

The development of requirements specific to the devices should be undertaken once the equipment to be purchased has been established. The specific requirements together with the general specifications will form the core of the specification document for the tender. A specific requirement document should include the following information:
- Types and quantities of devices
- Types and quantities of accessories and spare parts
- Intended usage of the devices including the location and operational environment
- Functional, performance, and operational requirements of the devices
- Any other requirements that is specific to the items to be purchased.

1.1.3 Testing and Acceptance

An important stage of the acquisition process is accepting the technology. Acceptance is a landmark to allow the technology to be put into clinical use. It also triggers a number of events including payment, start of the warranty period, etc. Therefore, it is important that the conditions of acceptance and test criteria are clearly spelled out in the specifications. The specifications should be written such that each requirement is verifiable. Verification methods may include test, demonstrate, inspection, and analysis. Ambiguous statements should be avoided. For example, the requirement statement "the device should warm blood" should be written as "the device must warm blood to a temperature between 39 and 40° C"; and the statement "it should have a small footprint" should be written as "it must not occupy more than a space of 1 meter by 2 meters on the counter of the central nursing station." The facility should also ensure that staff and equipment are available to perform the requirement verification.

1.2 Request for Proposal

In general, preparation of the request for proposal (RFP) is the responsibility of the Purchasing Department. However, the Technology Acquisition Working Group (TAWG) plays an important

role in putting the pertinent information together. For example, the biomedical engineer in the TAWG, based on requirements from the users and other supporting groups, will develop the requirement specifications. The Purchaser will then develop the rest of the documents in the RFP. The draft RFP will be circulated to the members of the TAWG for review and modification. A signature/cover sheet should be attached to the draft RFP to make sure that all members have reviewed the document before it is finalized. A request for proposal to the vendors should include the following information:
- Cover letter
- Tender instructions
- Tender deadline
- Tender submittal
- Requirement specifications
- Statements of tender evaluation and acceptance criteria
- Terms and conditions
- Methods of payment

The RFP should also contain a statement to encourage vendors to submit alternative solutions to the listed specifications.

1.3 The Tendering Process

In general, the Purchaser is responsible to oversee the tendering process and to make sure that all pertinent information is supplied to all venders and that fair purchasing practice is followed. In essence, the tendering process consists of the following phases:
- Development of vendor short list
- Request for Proposals (RFP) sent out to vendors
- Receipt of return tenders (should be sealed and returned before the deadline)
- Opening of tenders (normally, late tenders will not be accepted)
- Any change in the RFP (e.g., change in requirements, quantities, etc.) that needs resubmission should be sent to all vendors through a tender document addendum.

For acquisition of low cost items, the tendering and RFP processes, which are stringent and time consuming, are deemed to be unnecessary. In such cases, a quotation request can be sent out to prospective suppliers and the returned quotations will be collected and evaluated. Nonetheless, the quotation request should spell out as much details as necessary to avoid omissions and arguments after the purchase order is awarded.

2 PREPURCHASE EVALUATIONS

2.1 Issues to be considered

In order to ensure that a medical device or a technology meets the requirements and is truly of value, careful analysis of the tender proposals is critical. The process of equipment prepurchase evaluation can reveal unacceptable performance of either the equipment or its related accessories or supplies before it becomes a problem of the facility. In addition, the vendor's support commitment and past performance are often evaluated.

The procedures and criteria for ranking vendor proposals are to be formulated and preferably finalized by the TAWG at the time when the tender specifications are under preparation. These evaluation procedures and decision criteria must be in place at the beginning of the selection process. It is important that all members of the TAWG (in which the clinical user should be a member) participate in the development. These procedures and criteria should specify such items as the composition of the review team (i.e., nursing, lab technicians, BME, etc.), the schedule of the evaluation, the evaluation methods and data to be collected, etc. The evaluation work can be simplified substantially by establishing evaluation criteria that have definitive answers (e.g., each item is graded as either a "Yes" or a "No," indicating whether or not it complies with the requirement). The final recommendation should base on the result of the evaluation. Members of the TAWG who are involved in prepurchase evaluation of these new devices or systems should be aware of the following factors:

2.1.1 Safety Factor

Safety should be the first screening criterion in the evaluation process. The safety issues used to determine equipment acquisition are:

Incidents–Confirmed events within the institution or through notification from hazard alerts that have caused or have the potential of causing injury that is related to the device under consideration (e.g., malfunction or design problems).

- *Poor Reliability*–The number of equipment failures and the amount of downtime.
- *Regulatory Prohibition*–Specific local, provincial, or federal codes may prohibit or restrict the use of certain devices.
- *Lack of Safety Features*–The device lacks critical safety features according to the current standards. This factor is evaluated with respect to the patient, the user, and others who may be affected in the environment. Standards documents such as those published by CSA, evaluation reports published in the ECRI's "Health Devices," and clinical trials by clinical personnel are used to ascertain whether or not deficiencies exist.
- *Medical Inadequacy*–The device does not perform its function in compliance with the current standard of care as determined by consensus documents (such as those provided by the American Academy of Pediatrics) or as determined in other documented sources.

2.1.2 Support Factor

Support issues relevant to equipment prepurchase evaluations are:
- *Product Support Termination*–The manufacturer or vendor ceased to provide accessories, parts, and service to support the product. The RFP should require the vendors to provide this information. This issue of the availability of in-house support and alternative sources of parts must also be taken into consideration.
- *Poor Support*–The manufacturer offers an unacceptable level of product support. This would include poor customer service or technical support, delayed shipment of parts, and inadequate service documentation.
- *Excessive Repair Costs*–The ratio of lifetime repair cost to acquisition cost is evaluated. The RFP should request the vendors to indicate the equipment maintenance cost and cost of major replacement items. It should also request the vendor to include a quotation of service contract so that maintenance expenses after the warranty period can be included in the operating budget.

2.1.3 Standardization Factor

Whenever possible, a hospital should try to standardize the technology within the facility. It is undesirable to have different makes and models of one type of equipment floating around in a hospital. For example, if a hospital has several makes of cardiac defibrillators in the Emergency Department, the time delay for a clinician to figure out how to operate a particular unit during an emergency procedure may decrease the chance for a successful resuscitation. The advantages of equipment standardization are listed below:

- Increased operation efficiency due to familiarity of the device.
- Decreased operating errors.
- Reduced training costs.
- Reduced the number of stocked replacement parts.
- Decreased acquisition costs through volume discounts.
- Ability to swap units from one area to another when needed.

Standardization of interface to allow communications between devices and the hospital information system is also an important consideration.

2.1.4 Cost Advantages of Replacing Equipment

In some situations, the operating cost of old medical technology can be very expensive. Tracking of maintenance costs and studying the potential costs and benefits of upgrading, replacing, or purchasing new technology should be done on a regular basis. Technology obsolescence due to age, design limitations, or poor reliability should also be considered.

2.1.5 Other Factors

In addition to safety and support issues, depending on the characteristics of the technology, there are other factors that may need to be considered in a prepurchase evaluation (e.g., what is the impact of technology down-time on patient care and cost?). Using a team approach can avoid missing some of these issues.

2.2 Technical Evaluation

A medical technology should be evaluated from three different angles: technical, clinical, and financial. The purpose of technical and clinical evaluations are to determine whether the proposed technology meets the functional and performance needs whereas the financial evaluation looks at the cost of the technology.

The in-house service provider (e.g., the biomedical engineering staff) in most cases performs the technical evaluation in the prepurchase evaluation process. Technical evaluation involves analyzing the performance of the device or system and the technical documentation. It is often beneficial to consult with other facilities that own the same technology to reveal any service problems. Technical evaluations include studying and testing the:

- compliance of the technology with specifications listed in the RFP
- environmental and utilities requirements
- system performance
- physical construction
- reliability
- overall quality
- maintainability
- safety
- compatibility with existing devices and systems
- service support availability and quality
- requirements of service training
- requirements of special service tools and software
- completeness and quality of service instructions

An evaluation form and procedures should be developed and the results documented. Figure 9–1 at the end of this chapter shows a general technical evaluation form for medical devices.

2.3 Clinical Evaluation

The best method to evaluate a medical device is by putting the device to use in its intended clinical environment. Each short listed device quoted by the vendors should be brought in, if possible, for an actual trial for a period of time, say two to three weeks. In the clinical evaluation, the users should look at:

- clinical performance
- ease of use and setup
- ergonomics
- special requirements
- cleaning, disinfecting, and sterilization procedures
- user support
- quality of vendor in-service training
- completeness and quality of operating manuals

In order to objectively evaluate the devices and maintain consistency in the evaluation. The TAWG should develop an evaluation form with procedures and criteria before the clinical trial. An example of a clinical evaluation form for a "Neonatal Monitor" appears at the end of this chapter (Fig. 9–2).

2.4 Financial Analysis

Instead of just focusing on the initial capital investment, the life cycle cost of the technology should be used in the financial analysis. Life cycle cost analysis facilitates the comparison of proposals with significant variations in initial costs and ongoing expenditures. A net present value (NPV) analysis looking into inflation, future cash flow, and foregone of investment opportunities should be performed. NPV is the total amount that a series of future payments is worth now. In a simple example, when one borrows money from a bank, the amount of money lent to the borrower is the present value of the future payments. In computing the NPV, the following costs should be captured from the tender proposal and included in the calculation:
- investment in planning and decision making
- initial capital investment
- facility renovation
- lifetime supplies and disposables
- human resources (initial and ongoing)
- training
- lifetime maintenance and repairs
- disposal
- income from reimbursement, resale, etc.

Below is an example to calculate the net present value of the capital and operating costs in a capital acquisition process of a surgical laser. The two spreadsheets show the total present value calculation of the surgical lasers from two suppliers, A and B. Note that if only the initial capital cost is considered, Laser B will the obvious choice (given the same performance). However, when considering the total present value of the investment over a period of five years, Laser A costs less than Laser B.

Net Present Value Lifecycle Cost Analysis of Surgical Laser Acquisition
Laser A

	Initial Capital	*Year 1*	*Year 2*	*Year 3*	*Year 4*	*Year 5*
Laser	$80,000					
Accessories	$10,000					
Disposable		$4,500	$4,725	$4,961	$5,209	$5,470
Facility	$5,000					
Training	$2,500	$3,000				
Service			$10,000	$10,500	$11,550	$13,283
Other Support		$800	$840	$882	$926	$972
Total	$97,500	$8,300	$15,565	$16,343	$17,685	$19,725
NPV of $1 discounted at 5%	$1	$0.952	$0.907	$0.864	$0.823	$0.784
NPV	$97,500	$7,905	$14,118	$14,118	$14,550	$15,455
Total Present Value	**$163,645**					

Net Present Value Lifecycle Cost Analysis of Surgical Laser Acquisition
Laser B

	Initial Capital	*Year 1*	*Year 2*	*Year 3*	*Year 4*	*Year 5*
Laser	$60,000					
Accessories	$12,000					
Disposable		$8,000	$8,400	$8,820	$9,261	$9.724
Facility	$5,000					
Training	$2,500	$3,000				
Service			$12,000	$12,600	$13,860	$15,939
Other Support		$1,200	$1,260	$1,323	$1,389	$1,459
Total	$79,500	$12,200	$21,660	$22,743	$24,510	$27,122
NPV of $1 discounted at 5%	$1	$0.952	$0.907	$0.864	$0.823	$0.784
NPV	$79,500	$11,619	$19,646	$19,646	$20,165	$21,251
Total Present Value	**$171,827**					

2.5 Matrix Decision Chart

A set of clearly defined evaluation criteria will facilitate the decision process by focusing on the needs and benefits rather than relying on emotional perception. It was mentioned that the criteria for selection should be determined early in the acquisition process. The criteria must be derived from the defined needs and specifications and form the basis of the technical and clinical evaluations. The results of the evaluations and the financial analysis of every proposal are to be entered into a matrix decision chart. The matrix decision chart is to be designed such that the people involved in the process can objectively record the findings. These results should, as far as possible, be slotted into quantitative scales. Each criterion in the chart should be weighed according to its significance in the overall picture. Again, these weighing factors should be determined together with the evaluation criteria at the early stage of the acquisition process. These quantitative results and the weighing factors will yield a total score for each proposal. The decision matrix will then become an objective tool for the TAWG to draw the final decision.

The ECRI CADH model is an example of such a matrix decision chart. Similar charts can be custom developed from a spreadsheet program such as Microsoft Excel or Lotus 123.

Below is an example of a matrix decision chart for an infusion pump evaluation. In this example, the requirements in the specifications are translated into evaluation criteria in the chart. Weights are given to each requirement according to its relative importance. The result is given a "1" if the answer satisfies the requirement and a "0" otherwise. The score for each requirement is equal to the product of the result and the weight (high weight=10, medium=5, low=1). For example, if the result is "favorable" and the weight is "medium," the score will be 1 x 5 = 5. PUMP C has the highest total score in this example and hence should be the most favorable choice. Note that the score calculation did not take into account the cost of ownership of the pumps. The decision should be obvious that PUMP C has the lowest life cycle cost, otherwise the TAWG should analyze all factors and come up with a recommendation.

Infusion Pumps Decision Matrix

Criteria	Weight	Alternatives		
		PUMP A	*PUMP B*	*PUMP C*
List Price	....	$6,300	$6,225	$5,625
Typical Discount Range	....	15%to64%	53%to56%	15%to64%
Warranty Period	Medium	One year	One year	Two years
IV Set Type	....	Not specified	Not Specified	Not specified
Separate Lines for Drug Delivery	High	Yes	Yes	Yes (single Channel)
Event, Error, and Pump Setting Log	Medium	Yes	Yes (limited)	Yes
Ramping	Low	Manual Titration	Manual Titration	Manual Titration
Nurse Call	Medium	Optional	Optional	Yes
Anti-Free flow Protection	Medium	Yes	Yes	Yes
Piggybacking	Medium	Yes	Yes	Yes
Flow Range	....	1 to 999.9	1 to 9,999	0.1 to 999
Syringe Delivery	Low	Yes	No	Yes
Drug-Dose Calculation	High	No	No	Yes
Weight, kg (lbs.)	....	5.9 (13)	5.3 (11.6)	6.4 (14)
Front Panel Lockout	Medium	Yes	No	Yes
Number of Channels	....	2	1	2
Currently Using Manufacturer's Pumps	Medium	No	No	Yes
Hazards and Recalls	Medium	Yes	Yes	Yes
Normalized SCORE (scale: 1 to 10)		5.2	4.2	9.2*
RANKING		2	3	1

To calculate the score:

Weight: High = 10, Medium = 5, Low = 1

Maximum total score = 62 in 12 categories (with weight factors)

The total score of PUMP C (3rd column) would be: $5+10+1+5+5+5+1+10+5+5+0 = 57$

Normalized Score = $57/62 = 9.2$

3 MAKING THE AWARD

After making the selection, an award has to be issued to acquire the technology. A purchase order (PO) or purchase contract document is prepared and signed by the vendor and the facility to form a contractual agreement. This contract document should be prepared by the Purchasing Department and reviewed by the TAWG to avoid omissions. The purchase contract document must cover all terms and conditions that have been agreed upon by the vendor and the facility. Once the contract is issued, a copy should be sent to the user department and the Biomedical Engineering Department (or the in-house service provider). The requirements in the purchase contract will be used to guide the incoming inspection and subsequent training and maintenance activities. It will also serve as a legal binding document in case any dispute arises between the vendor and the health care facility.

3.1 Purchase Contract Document

The purchase contract document integrates equipment performance, installation requirements, after sales services, and any condition of sales. Most facilities have a standard set of contract conditions that covers the common subjects. For a straightforward purchase, the RFP and the responses or simply the quotation from the successful vendor can be attached and referred to in the standard purchase contract document. In other cases, a special purchase contract will need to be developed. The most straightforward approach to prepare the contract is by listing and modifying the requirements in the RFP taking into account the responses from the vendor and any amendments made in the tender process. The purchase contract document should address the following:
- model and quantities of the devices
- model and quantities of accessories and supplies
- delivery and installation requirements
- codes, standards, and approval requirements
- acceptance criteria and testing procedures
- clinical and service training
- software licensing and future updates
- documentation (both operation and service)

- user and technical support
- warranty conditions
- spare parts and service
- payment, price protection, penalty and cancellation clauses
- schedule of events including delivery, commissioning, payments, etc.

Quite often, the tender document returned from the vendor is included as an appendix to form the purchase contract package.

3.2 Commissioning and Acceptance

All medical devices and technologies must be inspected and tested before they are put into clinical use. It is necessary to evaluate incoming equipment with respect to the device performance and specifications according to the vendor's data sheets. All applicable test procedures and acceptance criteria should be spelled out in the purchase contract. The list should include:

- What is to be tested and according to which standards and procedures?
- Who is going to perform the tests? The vendor, in-house staff, or third-party contractors?
- Who is responsible to document the tests?
- What are the criteria for acceptance?
- When will the warranty start?
- Who is responsible for the cost of commissioning?
- What are the consequences of noncompliance?

Readers should refer to earlier chapters for a more in-depth discussion of the incoming inspection and acceptance processes.

TECHNICAL EVALUATION

REQUESTING DEPARTMENT: _____ P.O. NUMBER: _____

DEVICE DESCRIPTION: _____ INTENDED AREA OF USE: _____

MANUFACTURER: _____ VENDOR: _____

MODEL/PART NUMBER: _____ SERIAL/LOT NUMBER: _____

	EXCELLENT		AVERAGE		POOR	
QUALITY OF DESIGN AND ASSEMBLY:	A	B	C	D	E	N/A
EASE OF USE:	A	B	C	D	E	N/A
SERVICEABILITY:	A	B	C	D	E	N/A
OPERATING MANUAL:	A	B	C	D	E	N/A
SERVICE MANUAL:	A	B	C	D	E	N/A
USER IN-SERVICE SUPPORT:	A	B	C	D	E	N/A
TECHNICAL SERVICE SUPPORT:	A	B	C	D	E	N/A

QUALITATIVE COMMENTS _____

_____

CERTIFICATION: LABELING: _____   RISK CLASS: _____

SAFETY TEST: PASSED _____   FAILED _____

SERVICE TRAINING: DEFINITELY REQUIRED _____   REQUIRED _____
                    NOT REQUIRED _____

SPECIAL TROUBLE SHOOTING/REPAIR TOOLS: _____

_____

PERFORMANCE: _____

_____

OVERALL COMMENTS: _____

_____

_____

EVALUATED BY: _____   DATE: _____   TIME: _____ Hr.

Figure 9–1. General Technical Evaluation Form for Medical Devices.

CLINICAL EVALUATION

DEVICE DESCRIPTION:___Neonatal Monitor___   INTENDED AREA OF USE: __SCN__

MANUFACTURER:_____   VENDOR: _____

MODEL/PART NUMBER:_____   SERIAL/LOT NUMBER: _____

	EXCELLENT	AVERAGE	POOR
EASE OF USE AND SET UP			
ECG:	A	B	C
RESPIRATION:	A	B	C
PULSE OXIMETRY:	A	B	C
QUALITY OF WAVEFORM DISPLAY:	A	B	C
READABILITY OF NUMERIC DISPLAY:	A	B	C
READABILITY OF ALARM SETTINGS:	A	B	C
CLARITY OF AUDIBLE ALARM:	A	B	C
CLARITY OF VISUAL ALARM:	A	B	C
PORTABILITY:	A	B	C
PULSE OXIMETER SENSOR			
STAYS WELL ON PATIENT:	A	B	C
IMMUNE TO ARTIFACTS:	A	B	C
OVERALL RATING:	A	B	C

OTHER COMMENTS: _____

_____

DO YOU RECOMMEND PURCHASING THIS UNIT?   YES _____ NO _____

EVALUATED BY: _____   DATE: _____

Figure 9–2. Clinical Evaluation Form for a "Neonatal Monitor."

Chapter 10

TECHNOLOGY REPLACEMENT

The last phase of the technology life cycle deals with the replacement and retirement of medical technology. No medical devices can be used forever; there is always an end to the useful life of a particular device or system. The technology life cycle begins after a new one has replaced the old technology (see Fig. 10–1). The life cycle of modern medical technology tends to span from a period of five to ten years. In this chapter, we will look at some criteria to determine whether or not to replace or to keep a medical technology. Different approaches to dispose of retired technology will also be discussed.

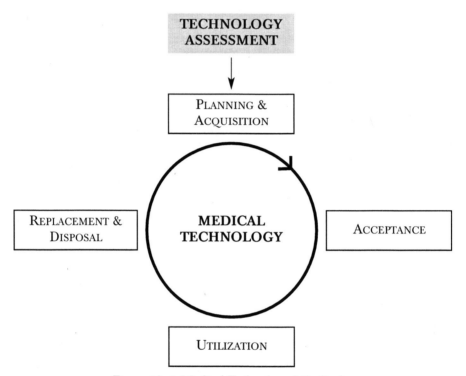

Figure 10–1. Medical Technology Life Cycle.

1 REASONS FOR TECHNOLOGY REPLACEMENT

Remember our car example in Chapter 2. In general, there are only two reasons for an individual to buy a new vehicle: either to have an additional vehicle or to replace an existing one. There are many possible reasons to replace the existing vehicle. The needs of the owner and the condition of the existing vehicle are some examples.

Similar reasons apply to the replacement of medical technology in a health care facility. The following questions are usually asked when considering medical technology replacement:

1. Does the technology meet the "standard of care"?
2. Is the technology obsolete?
3. Has it been replaced by a new or improved technology?
4. Is the frequency of failure and downtime excessive?
5. Is the technology expensive to maintain?
6. Is the replacement financially justifiable?
7. How are we going to finance the new technology?
8. What are we going to do with the retired technology?

These questions can be grouped into three categories: substandard of care and technology obsolescence, maintenance problems, and financial considerations.

1.1 Sub-standard of Care and Obsolescence

1.1.1 Substandard of Care

Standard of care refers to the acceptability of common practice. Safety violation is a primary reason to retire a medical technology. A hospital should, on a high priority, stop using and replace a medical device immediately if it is deemed to pose unjustifiable risk on patients or staff.

The advancement of medical technology has helped to raise the standard of care. For example, ECG arrhythmia detection, which was only used in highly acute care areas 15 years ago, is now a standard feature in all critical care physiological monitors. This is a direct result of the improvement and cost reduction in microprocessor technology. On the other hand, the risk of legal liability will increase if a health care facility is not using monitors with arrhythmia detection capability (substandard medical devices) in acute are areas.

1.1.2 Technology Obsolescence

A technology becomes obsolete when there is a another better alternative to serve the same purpose. For example, genetic therapy may one day eliminate the need to perform some medical procedures.

In recent years, the availability of new improved technology has catalyzed many technology replacements. Advancement in medical technology is also an enabling factor to raise the standard of care. Issues such as safety, reliability, clinical outcome, and cost often trigger development of new technologies and improvement to existing technologies. Infusion controllers are an example of a technology made obsolete by an improved technology—the infusion pumps. The availability of new and improved technology is perhaps the primary reason for technology replacement in developed countries.

Another reason for technology obsolescence is the termination of manufacturer's support, which will be discussed in the next section.

1.2 Maintenance Problems

1.2.1 Poor Reliability

Reliability is critical for medical technology. Many medical procedures cannot tolerate failure. An inaccurate or malfunctioning device can lead to incorrect diagnosis and subsequent mal-treatment. Clinicians may ignore a genuine alarm if they have lost confidence on a frequently failed or inaccurate device. Sometimes it is better off to remove such a device or system altogether.

1.2.2 Excessive Downtime

Frequent failure and lengthy downtime will decrease the availability of a technology and can cause cancellation of medical procedures. In additional, patients may not be treated promptly and properly. The hospital may have to turn away patients and result in loss of revenue. If a situation persists, the hospital will have to acquire additional spare equipment to cope with the downtime.

1.2.3 Lack of Service and Replacement Parts

Technical support is vital for effective and reliable operation of medical technology. Local support is desirable to provide fast service response. Delay to obtain replacement parts (e.g., parts need to be shipped from overseas) can increase the downtime of the equipment. In many countries, the manufacturers, by law, must notify their customers if they have decided to discontinue their products, which implies that maintenance and replacement parts will no longer be available. Some manufacturers may guarantee to continue their supply of replacement parts for a certain length of time after the last production run. A hospital must plan to replace the device when it has received such notification from the device manufacturer.

1.3 Financial Considerations

1.3.1 Maintenance Cost

Usually when a device gets older, the cost of maintenance will increase. Similar to a vehicle, parts (especially moving parts) will need to be serviced or replaced due to wear and tear. Manufacturers of ventilators and renal dialysis machines recommend that their devices have major overhauls according to the hours of usage. Such overhauls include parts replacement (often expensive) and operational verification inspections. It is not uncommon that replacing an ailing medical technology with a new one can achieve substantial savings.

1.3.2 Operating Cost

Operating cost comprises of the cost of labor to operate the device, the cost of supplies or consumables, and the cost of utilities. Digital radiography can improve the work flow so that the same number of staff in the same period of time can handle more patients. This results in an increase in operational efficiency (lower cost per X-ray). Replacing devices that use less expensive supplies can often achieve immense savings. For example, a hospital using 200 infusion sets a day will save $146,000 per year by replacing the old pumps with newer ones using cheaper sets that cost $2 less per set. Although it may not be a significant amount when compared to other costs, newer technology is usually more efficient, more reliable, and has less demands on electricity, water, or gases.

1.3.3 Loss of Revenue

A hospital will have to turn away patients when its CT scanner is not functional. Patients may be attracted to a hospital because of its state-of-the-art technology. These are financial issues that need to be addressed in the technology replacement strategy.

1.3.4 Patient Length of Stay

Critical care beds and operating room time are expensive in a hospital. Reducing the operating room time or decreasing the patient length of stay in a hospital may more than offset the cost of acquiring a new technology. Key-hole surgeries, using video endoscopes and special surgical tools, have turned many inpatient procedures that previously required lengthy hospital stay into outpatient day procedures. This is a good example to show how technology can reduce cost and improve efficiency in health care.

2 REPLACEMENT MANAGEMENT STRATEGY

2.1 Tracking Life-cycle Cost and Service History

The previous section discussed the importance of paying attention to the financial aspect when considering technology replacement. The life cycle cost of an existing technology can be calculated only if there is a tracking mechanism in place. The initial acquisition cost, including capital and installation, can often be obtained from the purchasing records. The cost of supplies or disposables may be estimated from the materials management archives. The on-going maintenance, as well as training expenses, can only be accounted for if all the work orders and service information were recorded. In order to track the operating cost of a technology, all support-related costs including labor, parts, and training expenses should be documented.

A computerized hospital equipment management program can provide service history and up-to-date information of the total service cost of a technology. From these data, one can estimate future service requirements that form part of the rationale to determine whether to keep or replace the technology in the hospital. Service histories, such as the frequency of failure and amount of downtime, are useful for capital equipment replacement planning. The service history can also indicate the serviceability of a similar model of medical device or represent the reliability of a product from a particular manufacturer. When properly documented and compiled, the above mentioned information can be useful in the facility-wide planning and acquisition process.

2.2 Replacement Planning

Technology replacement should be an integral component of technology planning. The expected life span of a technology needs to be factored into the life-cycle cost of the acquisition process. Technology replacement planning often falls into one of the following categories:

2.2.1 On Demand

When existing medical technology becomes unsafe, obsolete, or beyond economical repair, it will need to be replaced. A sudden catastrophic technology failure will create an unplanned financial burden on the health care facility. An effective medical technology management program with a good maintenance tracking mechanism will often be able to detect the onset of such failure.

2.2.2 Following the Capital Budget Cycle

Replacement of medical technology should be included in the multi-year capital plan based on the expected life span of the technologies. The plan should be reviewed periodically along with such information as projected clinical needs, service information, and trends in the standard of practice.

2.2.3 Following the Technological Life Cycle

A properly designed and implemented hospital equipment management system captures all the service history and maintenance expenditures of the technology. Periodic review of such information can trend the failure rates and provide an estimation of the future maintenance cost. Such information may be combined with other factors to adjust the priorities in technology replacement planning.

3 TECHNOLOGY RETIREMENT

3.1 Destinies of Retired Medical Technology

When a medical technology is retired and taken out of service, its destiny may fall into one of the following categories:
- Trade in (i.e., it will become the property of the new equipment supplier)
- Sell to others
- Use as spare or backup in the facility
- Scavenge for parts
- Donate to developing or third-world countries
- Put into storage
- Scrap and dispose of

3.2 Precautions when Disposing of Medical Devices

Both "trade in" and "sell to others" can recover some of the acquisition cost of the old technology and hence may partially offset the purchase cost of the new technology. However, in some countries like Canada, under the medical devices regulations, reselling or even donating a functional medical device makes the hospital become a medical device vendor. The hospital will then assume the liability as a medical device vendor. Therefore, it may not be worthwhile to resell retired medical devices unless it is of significant value. On the other hand, in some countries, there are for-profit companies whose businesses are to purchase retired medical devices, refurbish them, and resell them for a profit. Some nonprofit organizations will take donated medical devices, refurbish them, and then donate them to developing or third-world countries. A hospital will have to consider the condition of the device, the local regulations, and the hospital policies to determine which approach to take in disposing of its retired medical inventory.

Chapter 11

OVERVIEW OF STANDARDS
AND REGULATIONS

1 STANDARDS

The International Organization for Standardization (ISO) defines standards as "documented agreements containing technical specifications or other precise criteria to be used consistently as rules, guidelines, or definitions of characteristics, to ensure that materials products, process and services are fit for their purpose."

1.1 The Purpose of Standards

Imagine the situation when you are traveling in a foreign country and trying to use your credit card but find out that the card reader is not compatible to read your credit card. Fortunately, credit card companies have standardized on the format and information on the credit cards so that cardholders can use their cards wherever they go. On the other hand, the letters or documents that you received from the U.K. will most likely not fit your letter file folder. This is because the U.K. letter paper size is different from the standard A4 letter paper that used in North America. Although we may not be aware of it, standards play an important part of our daily life. Standards are written and published for the following three reasons:

1. Define the specifications or requirements of a product or service
2. Ensure safety and minimum performance of products and services
3. Facilitate compatibility among products and services from different manufacturers or suppliers

A "CE" marking on a medical device indicates that the product has achieved a satisfactory level of safety according to the appropriate directives and thus may be marketed throughout the European community. As medical products are being marketed worldwide, a manufacturer therefore needs to ensure that its product development and manufacturing processes are in compliance with the standard requirements of all the countries where the products are sold.

1.2 Types of Standards

Standards can fall into three categories:

1.2.1 Consensus or Voluntary Standards

Consensus or voluntary standards are those developed under the consensus process where manufacturers, users, consumers, and government come together voluntarily in open public sessions. Examples of such are the IEEE Standards. Most standards fall into this category.

1.2.2 Regulatory (or Mandatory) Standards

Regulatory (or mandatory) standards are those required by the laws, such as the Canadian Electrical Codes enacted by the Canadian Government. Manufacturers must manufacture their products in compliance with the Codes in order to have their electrical devices legally sold in Canada. Regulatory standards may be developed by a government agency or adopted from voluntary standards.

1.2.3 Proprietary Standards

Proprietary standards are developed either by a company for its own internal use or by an association for use by its members. They can serve as a basis for voluntary or mandatory standards if the appropriate exposure is given and if there is consensus reached among all parties. An example of a proprietary standard is the EIA Interim Standard IS-3-D produced by the Electronic Industries Association.

1.3 Standards Development

1.3.1 Standard Development Bodies

Special interest groups or voluntary associations (e.g., IEEE in the US, CSA in Canada, IEC in Europe) may develop standards. Usually, there is only one official standard organization in a country (e.g., the CEN in Europe, ANSI in the U.S., and SCC in Canada) to coordinate and accredit standards development bodies as well as to represent the country in the international standardization organizations. An official standard organization would have the authority to endorse a standard as a national standard in its country. The official standard organizations in the United States, Canada, and Europe and their web sites are listed in Table 11–1.

The three major international standardization organizations are also listed in Table 11–1. In general, ITU covers work in the field of telecommunications, IEC in the field of electrical and electronics and ISO covers the rest.

Table 11-1

MAJOR NATIONAL AND INTERNATIONAL
STANDARDIZATION ORGANIZATIONS

Standard Organization	Web Site
American National Standards Institute (ANSI)	www.ansi.org
Standards Council of Canada (SCC)	www.scc.ca
European Community for Standardization (CEN)	www.cenorm.be
Japanese Standards Association (JSA)	www.jsa.or.jp
International Telecommunication Union (ITU)	www.itu.int
International Electro-technical Commission (IEC)	www.iec.ch
International Organization for Standardization (ISO)	www.iso.ch

1.3.2 Standard Numbering Format

Standards are usually identified by an alphanumeric numbering system. The leading alphabets indicate the standard body that published the standard (e.g., CSA, AAMI, EN, BS). The middle alphanumeric numbers identify the specific standard and the trailing numbers record the year in which the standard was finalized. Instead of reinventing the wheel, many standard bodies will adopt standards developed by another standard body. The following three examples illustrate the format of standard numbering:

1. "ASTM F1452–92: Standard Specification for Minimum Performance and Safety Requirements for Components and Systems of Anesthetic Gas Monitors" is published by the American Society for Testing and Materials (ASTM) in 1992 with the standard identification number F1452.

2. "ANSI/AAMI EC53–1995: ECG Cables and Wires" is a standard developed by the Association for the Advancement of Medical Instrumentation (AAMI) with an identification number EC53. It is adopted as an American national standard by the American National Standards Institute (ANSI) in 1995.

3. "CAN/CSA–ISO/IEC 9316–97: Information Technology– Small Computer System Interface–2" is a standard developed by the International Electro-technical Commission (IEC) with identification number IEC 9316. It is adopted as an international standard by the International Organization for Standardization (ISO) with identification number ISO/IEC

9316. This same standard is in turn adopted by the Canadian Standards Association as a CSA Standard (standard identification number CSA–ISO/IEC 9316). After being approved as a national standard of Canada by the Standard Council of Canada (SCC) in 1997, it is given a standard identification number of CAN/CSA–ISO/IEC 9316–97.

1.3.3 Standard Development Process

Standard development is usually triggered by needs such as a new technology. A request is often forwarded to a standard development body by a consumer organization, trade or industry association, or a government department. A recognized standard development body usually coordinates the development of a standard to ensure that the process is transparent and unbiased. A technical committee is then struck to consider the views of all participants and develop the details of the standard. The standard technical committee is structured to include experts as well as to represent diverse interests. Rather than using a simple majority-of-vote process, a committee in general develops standard details by a consensus process that encourages substantial agreement among committee members. The following is the usual sequence of events that occur in standard development:

1. Review request
2. Form a technical committee
3. Draft standard
4. Seek input from public/interested parties
5. Review input/comments
6. Revise draft
7. Seek input on revised draft
8. Second review
9. Approve standard
10. Publish standard
11. Periodical review and revision

When developing a standard, the standard technical committee needs to keep in mind that the standard should be based on scientific facts and experience and that, when completed, will benefit the whole community affected within the scope of the standard.

1.3.4 Standard Conformance

The primary method to assess conformity of a product to a standard is by direct testing. Testing is performed in different phases of the device development and utilization cycle according to the criteria laid down by the standards.

A process can be audited and certified to conform to a relevant standard by a certification agent or auditor. For example, a medical device manufacturer may recruit a notified body (certified auditor) to audit its quality management system according to ISO13485/ISO9001 standards (in Canada or Europe) or the CGMP (in the United States).

Health care facilities are often audited or accredited by their own professional association. The accreditation process involves assessing the facility against a set of service standards. An example of such service standards is the "Clinical Engineering Standards of Practice" published by the Canadian Medical and Biological Engineering Society (www.cmbes.ca).

1.3.5 Global Harmonization

As mentioned earlier, one of the main purposes of standards development is to facilitate compatibility among products and services from different manufacturers or suppliers. Having a set of global medical device standards and regulations will promote international trade, ensure device compatibility, facilitate technological development, provide more choices for the consumers as well as reduce production costs.

In 1992, a voluntary group of representatives from national medical device regulatory authorities formed the Global Harmonization Task Force (GHTF). The founding countries included Australia, Canada, the European Union, Japan, and the United States. The purpose of the GHTF is, according to its summary statement, "to encourage convergence in regulatory practices related to ensuring the safety, effectiveness/performance and quality of medical devices, promoting technological innovation and facilitating international trade, and the primary way in which this is accomplished is via the publication and dissemination of harmonized guidance documents on basic regulatory practices." Guidance documents on regulatory practices published by the GHTF can be found in the GHTF web site (www.ghtf.org).

2 REGULATIONS

2.1 Acts, Regulations and Guidance Documents

Regulations are, in most cases, standards that are made mandatory by a government. Regulations are established to serve one or more of the following purposes:
- To ensure devices sold and used are safe
- To make sure products and services are consistent
- To facilitate correction and recall actions by manufacturers
- To ensure problems are reported

Acts or statutes contain general statements covering a wide scope of applications, whereas regulations are derived from the relevant acts or statues to provide specifics and details. In Canada, the Canadian Food and Drugs Acts established by the Parliament provides the legal power for the Medical Devices Regulations to regulate the sales and use of medical devices.

Acts and regulations are legal documents. Guidance documents are often written in plain language to explain the regulations. For example, "The Electric Code Simplified" is a guidance document to interpret and provide specific details to the "Canadian Electric Code."

2.2 Medical Device Regulations

The rapid proliferation of technology in health care in the past few decades has a major impact on the practice of medicine. The concerns of medical device safety and efficacy have precipitated in the development of medical device regulatory systems in many countries. Despite the efforts to harmonize medical device standards and regulations, regulatory systems are still different from one country to another. Nonetheless, they all share the same philosophy–to minimize risk.

2.2.1 Device Classification

In order to minimize the unnecessary effort that device manufacturers have to put in to reduce risk, many countries require a classification system on medical devices based on the risk level of the device under use. The criteria for risk assessment usually include:
- the degree of invasiveness
- the location and duration of the contact
- the extensiveness and effect of device to the subject

Higher-risk medical devices require more stringent control, whereas lower-risk devices have less regulatory requirements to reduce costs. For example, the Canadian Medical Devices Regulations (1998) separates medical devices into four risk classes, with Class I representing the lowest risk, to Class IV representing the highest risk. Some examples of devices for each class are shown below:

Class I–band-aids, ultrasound gel

Class II–contact lenses, latex gloves

Class III– indwelling catheters, IV bags

Class IV–pacemakers, defibrillators

Details of the Regulations can be found in the Health Canada web site (www.hc-sc.gc.ca). The European medical directive (Class I, IIa, IIb, III) and the U.S. FDA (Class I, II, III) have similar classification systems.

2.2.2 Regulatory Control

The terms premarket review and postmarket surveillance/vigilance are often used in medical devices regulations. For our discussion, we separate regulatory control into three stages: premarket review, sales control, and postmarket surveillance/vigilance. Premarket review covers the development and production phases of medical devices and is sometimes referred to as product control. Sales control covers the marketing and sales activities. Postmarket surveillance/vigilance covers the use and disposal of the devices. Figure 11–1 summaries the various stages of regulatory control.

Premarket Review

Premarket review covers the development, production, and labeling of the medical device to ensure that it is safe, effective, and performs according to its design under the stated operational conditions.

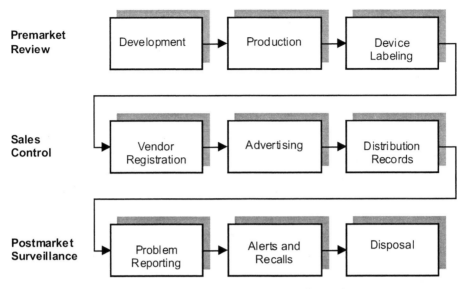

Figure 11–1. Stages of Regulatory Control.

The degree of scrutiny for premarket review is usually depending on the Risk Class of the device. Accurate labeling is required for all medical devices irrespective of their risk classifications. The premarket review requirements in the process of medical device development and production will be discussed in more details in the next chapter. The manufacturer of a medical device is required to clearly label the device's intended use and provide performance and safety information as well as users and maintenance instructions.

Sales Control

In Canada, under the Medical Devices Regulations, all distributors of medical devices are required to register with Health Canada (to obtain an Establishment License). The "Establishment" must attest that procedures are in place including: distribution of records, complaint handling, mandatory problem reporting, recalls, handling, storage, and corrective action. Furthermore, misleading and false advertisements are prohibited. Similar requirements exist in the U.S. and the European Union.

Postmarket Surveillance/Vigilance

While premarket review ensures that the products are designed to be safe, effective, and reliable, it may not be able to foresee operational problems especially from misuse. Postmarket surveillance/vigilance serves to complement the premarket review process. According to the Global Harmonization Task Force (GHTF), "Vigilance" refers to the routine monitoring of the product in accordance with national processes and procedures while "surveillance" refers to postmarket activities specifically invoked to confirm or refute predefined product-associated outcomes. The registration or licensing process under sales control requires the distributor to be responsible for postmarket surveillance/vigilance. It requires manufacturers and distributors to setup a system to track and investigate operating problems and incidents as well as to recall and modify defective items. In addition, some government authorities such as the U.S. FDA mandate users to report device-related problems.

2.2.3 Quality Systems Requirements

Most regulatory authorities require medical device companies to maintain a documented quality system in compliance to a specific quality management standard. The benefits of a documented quality system include:
- Reduced development cost
- Improved communication
- Consistent and controlled production
- High quality, safe, and reliable product
- Reduced support cost
- Access to international markets

In the U.S., medical device companies are legally required to comply with the Quality System Regulation (21 CFR part 820), in Europe with EN46001 or EN46002, and in Canada with ISO13485/ISO9001 or ISO13488/ISO9002. These quality systems cover the development, purchasing, manufacturing, packaging, labeling, storage, installation, and servicing aspects of medical devices. Under these quality systems, activities and product performance and conformance to specifications are monitored; any deviations from device and process specifications and company policies are fed back into the system; a correction action protocol is used to improve performance and conformance.

Proof of compliance to the quality system is done through quality documents developed and kept by the company and audited by certification bodies. The document hierarchy of a documented quality system is shown in Figure 11–2.

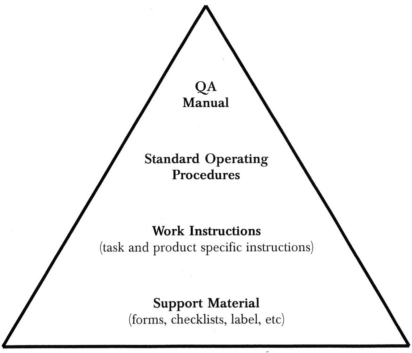

Figure 11–2. Hierarchy of a Documented Quality System.

Chapter 12

INTRODUCTION TO
MEDICAL DEVICE DEVELOPMENT

1 OVERALL LIFE CYCLE OF A TECHNOLOGY

The overall life cycle of a medical technology can be separated into three subcycles, as shown in Figure 12–1 with the output being passed from one subcycle to another. The acquisition and utilization subcycles have been discussed in detail in the earlier part of this book. In this chapter, we will look at the medical technology development subcycle.

So far, we have been studying the medical technology life cycle from the user's perspective. Although medical technology develop-

145

ment is not the focus of this book, this chapter provides a brief overview of the development process to complete the entire life-cycle discussion.

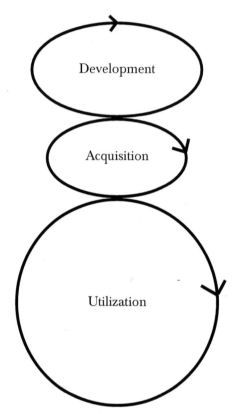

Figure 12–1. Medical Technology Life.

1.1 Technology Life Cycle–The Developer's Perspective

The life of a technology starts at a perceived need such as the need to measure blood glucose level for diabetic patients. A research team may come up with an idea to measure blood glucose level noninvasively by measuring the optical absorption of perspiration from the skin surface. This hypothesis may be verified by proof of concept experiments and eventually developed into a marketable product. The different stages of medical technology development are shown in Figure 12–2.

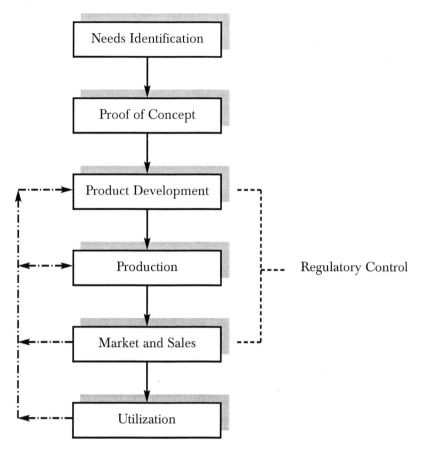

Figure 12–2. Process of Technology Development.

Market information in terms of enhancement and problems will be fed back into the development and production processes. Product development, production, market, and sales are subjected to regulatory control. In some jurisdictions, device problems identified by users are required to be reported to the manufacturers and local authorities. An overview of design assurance and risk management requirements and practices will be discussed in this chapter.

1.2 Market Cycle of a Medical Technology

The longevity of a medical technology depends on a number of factors:

- *Availability of a replacement technology*–the market share of a technology will diminish if there is a competitive product in the market, especially if the competitor is superior in performance or less expensive.

- *Availability of another more effective alternative technology*–the sales of a technology will be adversely affected if another technology with better clinical outcome is brought into the market. An example is the abandonment of using ultrasound lithotripsy to remove gall bladder stones when keyhole surgery becomes available.

- *Change of safety standards*–a product will cease to be used quickly if it is deemed unsafe by regulatory bodies or by the industry.

The life span of a technology in terms of its market volume can be separated into five periods. They are:

1. Introductory
2. Growth
3. Mature
4. Decline
5. Obsolescence

Figure 12–3 shows the volume of sales at different periods of the technology life span. In technology acquisition, it is important to understand at which period in its life span a technology is in to avoid acquiring a near-obsolete or premature technology.

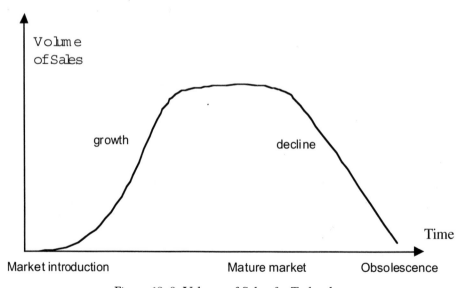

Figure 12–3. Volume of Sale of a Technology.

2 MEDICAL TECHNOLOGY DEVELOPMENT

From the medical technology producer's perspective, the technology life cycle consists of the following phases (note that this book has so far been focusing on the technology life cycle from the users' perspective):

1. Conceptualization
2. Research and feasibility study
3. Development
4. Manufacturing
5. Marketing and sales
6. Operation and technical support
7. Surveillance and vigilance
8. Obsolescence

Phases one to four are considered as premarket activities while six to eight are postmarket activities. The development phase is of particular interest to regulatory authorities due to the fact that it is a critical phase in determining the safety and reliability of the device. The U.S. FDA, in a study from 1983 to 1989, found that approximately 44 percent of the quality problems that let to voluntary recall actions were attributed to errors or deficiencies that were designed into particular devices and may have been prevented by adequate design controls. The following sections provide an overview of design assurance and risk management in medical device development.

2.1 Design Life Cycle

The development phase of a medical technology can be broken down into a number of separate activities with the output of one becoming the input to the next. This sequence of activities is often referred to as the design life cycle. The design life cycle is a structured approach which has been developed and refined by systems developers to design and build quality systems in view to increase efficiency, reduce cost, and improve reliability.

The Classic Waterfall model shown in Figure 12–4 has been used extensively in design assurance (there are other models used but will not be elaborated in this book). In this model, the output of each activity is the input of the next. The end-of-activity documents are reviewed and approved before the completion of the subsequent activity. Although the order of occurrence of the activities is fixed, to reduce development time, adjacent activities are allowed to time overlap thus allowing two of them to be running in parallel. Reviews are performed at different stages of the design by individuals outside the design team to look for obvious omissions and to ensure the design processes are followed. The output of the design life cycle is a set of production specifications to be transferred to the production floors.

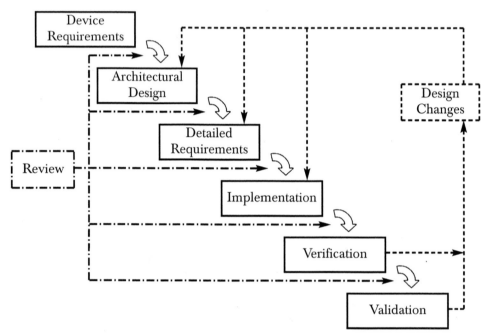

Figure 12–4. Classic Waterfall Model of Design Assurance.

2.2 Design History File

The design history file (DHF) is an important set of documents in quality assurance and regulatory submissions. Each activity in the design life cycle is documented and kept in the DHF. A DHF file is a compilation of the design history of a product, including its accessories, labeling, and packaging. It records the design process to show that plans were created, followed, and specifications were met. It also contains the results of the design reviews performed in the design life cycle.

3 RISK MANAGEMENT

3.1 The cost of hazard

Risk management in medical device development is an important process to ensure a safe and high-quality product. Risk management should be an integral part of the overall quality management program covering the entire device life cycle. We have looked at risk management from the user's perspective in earlier chapters. From the device developer's perspective, it is critical to be able to identify potential hazards as early as possible in the design life cycle. A potential hazard identified during the initial design of the product may require some engineering time to modify some design drawings. To mitigate a problem when the product is widely used in the market could incur a huge expense or even lead to litigations. Figure 12–5 shows the relative cost of hazard mitigation at different stages in the life span of a medical device. There were cases in which medical device companies were forced into bankruptcy because of safety problems not addressed in the development and production phases. An effective risk management program, especially starting at the initial design stage, will mini-

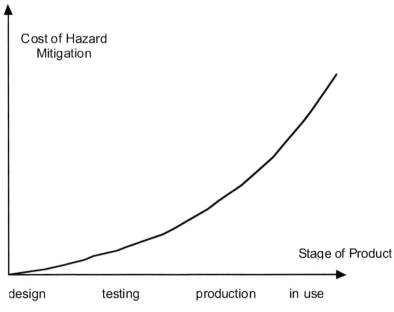

Figure 12–5. Cost of Device Hazard.

mize the occurrence of such problems. Interested readers should refer to the Standard ISO 14971:2000–application of risk management to medical devices.

3.2 Hazard Analysis

Hazard associated with a medical product may be due to its inherent design or caused by external factors such as inappropriate use (Fig. 12–6). Quite often, it is due to a combination of the above and may not be obvious to the designers in the development phase. A proactive approach in risk management encompasses the identification of potential hazards and the severity of harm as well as the analysis of their causes. Hazard identification needs a systematic study of the product including its operational environment and its intended use.

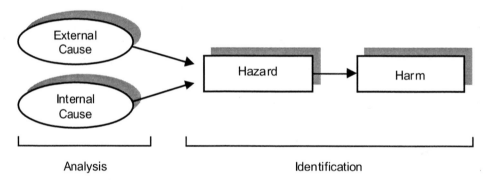

Figure 12–6. Risk Management.

Hazard analysis is the systematic evaluation of a device from the users' and patients' perspectives. Its purpose is to identify potential failure that could cause harm so that the design can be modified to avoid the problem. Figure 12–7 shows the principle of hazard evaluation. It measures the probability of occurrence of the hazardous situation and the severity of harm. A low probability and harmless situation will be tolerated while a highly probable and severely harmful situation will need mitigation actions such as a major product redesign. If we define risk R as the product of the probability of occurrence P and the severity of harm S (i.e., $R = P \times S$), the dotted line in the graph (Fig. 12–7) shows the locus of a constant risk level. If the dotted line is

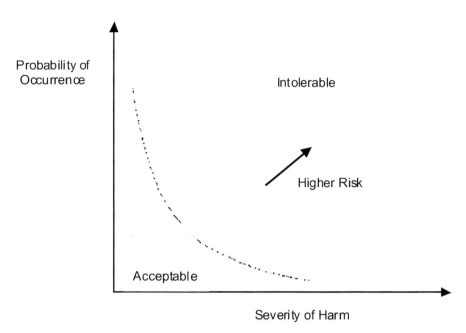

Figure 12–7. Hazard Analysis.

the limit of acceptable risk for a particular hazard, any situations falling on the right side of the dotted line are not acceptable and need to be mitigated.

3.2.1 Initial Hazard Analysis

Initial hazard analysis (IHA) is a qualitative approach to evaluate the possible harms and their severity associated with a device. IHA is often performed at an early stage of the design life cycle. Specifically, an IHA includes:

- Compilation of potential hazard list and the causes–these are potential harms and their causes with respect to users and patients.
- Assessment of risk–risk assessment involves identifying the severity (S) and the probability (P) of the hazard. A risk index (RI) for each hazard is then computed to determine the level of acceptance.
- Proposal of mitigate methods–based on the risk assessment, methods to mitigate the hazardous situations are identified.

Table 12–1 is an example of the IHA of a medical device. A severity scale of I to IV (e.g., I = least severe to IV = most severe) and a probability scale of A to D (A = least likely to happen, D = happens frequently) are used in this example. The risk index is determined from the combination of severity and probability. An example of risk index is shown in Table 12–2.

Table 12–1

EXAMPLE OF INITIAL HAZARD ANALYSIS

Hazard ID	Hazard	Cause	S	Mitigation	P	RI
H1	Injury caused by an electrical shock	Failure to limit voltage and/or energy stored in the device	II	Device designed to comply with IEC601-1, #15	A	2
H2	Injury caused by sharp edges	Faulty design or fabrication of mechanical components	III	Device designed to comply with EN60601-1 #23	B	5

Table 12–2

RISK INDEX TABLE

Probability of Occurrence	Severity Scale			
	IV	III	II	I
D	16	12	7	4
C	13	9	6	3
B	10	5	4	2
A	4	3	2	1

Risk Index	Acceptance Criteria
12 to 16	Unacceptable, must reduce risk
9 to 11	Undesirable, advisable to reduce risk
5 to 8	Acceptable, consider to reduce risk
1 to 4	Acceptable

3.2.2 Detailed Hazard Analysis

Detailed hazard analysis (DHA) uses the results of IHA as starting points to perform a detailed study of the cause and solution of the hazardous situation. Common methods used to perform DHA include

"Fault Tree Analysis" (FTA) and "Failure Mode and Effect Analysis" (FMEA).

1. FAULT TREE ANALYSIS. FTA is deductive and proceeds from the top down. It examines the hazard and locates the possible failures in the system that produced the hazard. FTA uses the information developed in the IHA as well as the device architecture and design. A potential hazard identified in the IHA is analyzed at the architectural level and eventually expanded to the root cause. Each level of the tree is broken down to lower level failures until the cause of the failure is found. Those who are interested to learn more about the process should read the standard "IEC61025 Fault Tree Analysis (FTA)".

2. FAILURE MODE AND EFFECT ANALYSIS. FMEA is inductive and proceeds from the bottom up. It is a method to understand the effect of component failures on hazards. It examines whether a single failure of a low-level component or a combinational failure of multiple components can cause failures in higher-level subsystems, and whether such failures can create a hazard. The standard "IEC60812 Analysis Techniques for System Reliability–Procedure for Failure Mode and Effects Analysis (FMEA)" provides more details on the process.

3.2.3 Timing of Hazard Analysis

Initial hazard analysis should be performed after the device requirements are specified and should be updated whenever there is a change in the requirements. FTA could start right after the architectural design is completed; the tree could be expanded when more details are unveiled. FMEA is best carried out after the device design is completed as it starts at the component level (bottom up).

As discussed earlier, hazard analysis should start as early as possible in the product development cycle. On the other hand, hazard analysis may also be applied to a device already in use in the field, although it will be very expensive to make field upgrades should design changes be required as a result of the analysis.

INDEX